th conception chronicles

the

uncensored truth

about sex,

love & marriage

when you're

TRYING

to get pregnant

Patty Doyle Debano
Courtney Edgerton Menzel
Shelly Dicken Sutphen

Health Communications, Inc.
Deerfield Beach, Florida

www.bcibooks.com

Library of Congress Cataloging-in-Publication Data

Debano, Patty Doyle, 1966-
    The conception chronicles : the uncensored truth about sex, love &
marriage when you're trying to get pregnant / Patty Doyle Debano,
Courtney Edgerton Menzel, Shelly Dicken Sutphen.
        p. cm.
    Includes bibliographical references.
    ISBN-13: 978-0-7573-0238-1
    ISBN-10: 0-7573-0238-6
    1. Conception—Popular works. 2. Fertility, Human—Popular works.
3. Infertility—Treatment—Popular works. 4. Human reproductive
technology—Popular works. 5. Infertility—Psychological aspects.
    I. Menzel, Courtney Edgerton, 1966- II. Sutphenn, Shelly Dicken, 1965-
III. Title.

RG133.D43 2005
18.1'78—dc26

                                                                2005040437

Publisher: Health Communications, Inc.
                3201 S.W. 15th Street
                Deerfield Beach, FL 33442-8190

Cover and Inside Chapter Openers design by Andrea Perrine Brower
Inside book design by Dawn Von Strolley Grove

For our husbands . . .
because what happened in the bedroom
didn't stay in the bedroom

Contents

Acknowledgments

It's hard to believe what started as three girlfriends doing what friends do best—chatting and e-mailing about life's challenges and experiences—has turned into this . . . a book! The steps between "Hey, this would be a great book" and the final result you are holding in your hands could not have been accomplished without the help and support of many people.

First, there are our husbands. Yes, they thought it would be great to share our most intimate experiences with the world—of course that was over a cold beer on vacation when they thought there wasn't a snowball's chance in hell it would ever happen. When we actually "sold" the idea, many a lesser man would have run for cover and insisted on editing rights to all things embarrassing. Not so, our men checked their modesty (and their pride) at the door so we could truly tell it like it was. Of course, everything takes more time than you expect. The many trips between New York, Chicago and California whittled into precious family time. Samantha, Connor and Maré, we hope you are too young to remember the soccer games and swimming lessons we missed along the way. If not, we're setting aside a portion of the book's proceeds to bribe your future forgiveness.

We'd like to give a big shout out to our families as well—it's no coincidence we've all included our maiden names on the cover. We are all lucky enough to have families who have offered their unwavering support not only for the book but also for the journey behind the book. Our parents have been a constant source of encouragement and love, and we only hope we can do half as well with our own children. Aside from the mushy stuff, our mothers have laughed at every story we've shared and acted as the FCC to censor the most graphic details from our conservative fathers. Thank you!!

Before we leave the family tree, we must acknowledge our brothers and sisters—you are the reason we are working so hard to build a family. Sure, our arms still hurt from punch bug, and we'll never forget the time you sent *Barbie* into space on your power rocket, but that's what it's all about . . . family. Kim, your cell phone bills prove you are the best sister in the world (actually, it's a tie with Leslie). Not only did you listen endlessly to fertility treatment options, but you offered a shoulder to cry on and provided laughs when they were needed most. DJ, as always, you came through with your creativity and contacts.

Of course, this book would not be a book without the help of our wonderful agent, Barbara Collins Rosenberg. Barbara was the first person without a genetic link to us who believed in this project. She took a chance to work with three "nobodies," and for this we thank her. Through Barbara's tenacity, we found Allison Janse— the greatest editor one could hope to work with. Not only did Allison "get it," she was one of us—having battled her own fertility issues. There was an instant connection, which made writing the book as much fun as it was work.

Last, but certainly not least, we want to thank all of our girlfriends who have cheered for us along the way and shared their own personal experiences for all the world to read. We count ourselves lucky to have such great women in our lives. Whether it's battling the minefields of fertility treatment or heading to Miami on a girls' weekend, it's great to have your girlfriends by your side.

Introduction

D o you remember the moment? The moment you knew you wanted to have a baby.

Some women are touched in a way they never knew possible when a stroller passes by carrying a chubby cheeked, angelic infant. For some, it's the heartrending pinkie clutch of a newborn niece who refuses to let go that stirs a dormant instinct. While for others, they just feel it in their hearts—they're ready.

It doesn't matter how or why you came to the decision; the point is you're here. You're trying to have a baby! Welcome to the Club —you're officially a TTC. We've taken to affectionately calling our girlfriends who've set out on the journey to motherhood TTCs (friends who are "Trying To Conceive").

Three Friends, Three Laptops and a Thing Called E-Mail

We—Shelly, Courtney and Patty—met in New York City fresh out of college when our biggest concerns were making it to work on time, finding knockoff couture fashions to match our entry-level salaries and meeting for our weekly Sunday brunch at the all-you-can-eat Chinese buffet.

Soon we were scattered across the world, married and trying our best to act like grown-ups. Courtney was the first to venture into motherhood. The minute she ordered a ginger ale on a girls' weekend in Puerto Rico, we knew she had an announcement to make. Nine months later she had a beautiful baby girl, and two years after that a bouncing baby boy.

Shelly was the next to start a family. While living in New Zealand, she gave birth to the cutest little Kiwi—a precious baby girl. Even though we didn't see each other often, our friendship remained solid across the miles. We did, however, have to make some minor adjustments. One day, Patty's husband opened the phone bill and screamed, "Our calling card was stolen!" After reviewing the bill more carefully, Patty had to admit that the total, as shocking as it was, was not the result of larceny but rather the legitimate highway robbery of international long-distance rates. This was the day we decided our primary means of communication would be e-mail.

We shared everything with each other (or so we thought). Nothing was off-limits—marital squabbles, career blunders, pie-in-the-sky dreams and our husbands' bad bathroom etiquette. But it wasn't until Patty felt the "baby urge" that we discussed Courtney's and Shelly's experiences trying to have a baby.

When Patty's plans for pregnancy were not falling into place as expected, she e-mailed Courtney and Shelly for advice. Patty was surprised to learn how long it took Courtney to get pregnant with her first child. They had never talked about the year Courtney spent testing her saliva each morning to see if she was ovulating or the anxiety Courtney and her husband, Dan, felt each month that passed without a pregnancy.

Why didn't we talk about it? We were the closest of friends, but Courtney consciously decided not to share her efforts with us or with anyone else for that matter. She went through twelve months of trying alone. Did she think what she was going through wasn't normal? Did she think we'd think less of her? Why didn't she share her struggle with her best friends?

Maybe it was because we hadn't stepped foot down the pregnancy path, and Courtney didn't think we'd be even remotely interested in hearing about the shades of blue you need to decipher on an ovulation stick or the details around saliva testing. However, the truth is that Courtney was simply embarrassed to admit getting pregnant was not as easy as she thought it would be.

Fertility Honesty

If you've just recently become a TTC ("Trying To Conceive" for those who aren't used to the acronym yet), you may wonder what the big secret is about trying to get pregnant: Why don't women talk about the problems they have trying to conceive? Since 9 million Americans seek help with their fertility issues each year, couldn't we all benefit from each other's trials and tribulations?

We asked ourselves these questions when we started to be candid about our own personal stories. As Patty struggled to conceive her first child, she found great comfort in the fact that her best friends understood her monthly disappointment and frustration. While Shelly didn't have any problem conceiving her first child, she had no idea how hard it would be trying for number two. Through the course of writing this book, Shelly's role shifted from that of supportive friend to a TTC herself, dealing with her own struggle to get pregnant.

We found that during the darkest days, a strong shoulder, a kind word and a lot of humor really helped soften the rough spots. We realized if we could help each other maybe there was a way to reach other women who were facing the same struggles alone. Once we came clean with our fertility struggles, we were amazed at how many of our friends had their own personal stories to share as well. They've been gracious enough to allow us to include their tales throughout this book. While intimate and at times embarrassing, these "Tales from the TTCs" are true. We've changed these women's names to preserve their marriages and the dignity of their unsuspecting husbands. That's how *The Conception Chronicles* came to be: what began as a series of e-mails and conversations among girlfriends evolved into this book. Our hope is that it's a friend you can turn to, to help you through those embarrassing, uncomfortable and sometimes outrageous moments that go along with trying to have a baby.

We wish you a short and speedy road to motherhood. But if you find you are confronted with some unexpected roadblocks, sharp curves or breathtaking drop-offs along the way, know that you are not alone. We've been there too.

chapter one

Practice Makes Perfect, Right?

Monday   Notes

- ~~Fill birth control prescription~~
- Fill prenatal vitamin prescription

Tuesday   Notes

- Check maternity leave policy with HR

Wednesday   Notes

- Pick up book of baby names

Pulling the Goalie

"**A**re you trying?" Unless you walked down the aisle pregnant, you should expect to be asked if you're trying to have a baby from the minute you get back from your honeymoon 'til the moment your belly is bulging.

Deciding to have a child is the single biggest decision you will ever make. No doubt, you have spent hours contemplating parenthood: Are we ready? Is this the right time? Is the house big enough? You've probably had some type of blueprint in place for your life, and up until this point, you've been the one in control. So naturally, as you think about starting a family, you assume having a baby will be under your control as well. You conveniently slot children into your master plan:

(1) Marriage
(2) Build career
(3) Find bigger apartment/buy house
(4) Travel
(5) Purchase beloved family dog
Insert Here → **First Child**
(6) Upgrade to roomier, dual–car seat capacity vehicle
Insert Here → **Second Child**
(7) Expand house
Insert Here → **Third Child (optional)**

Our parents, mothers in particular, may accuse us of overanalyzing the possibility of parenthood. According to Mom, in her day people just had kids and "it all worked out." But times have changed, and things today are much more complicated. You know you want children, but you have a long list of concerns about bringing a new life into this world. You worry about all the violence that exists close to and far away from home. What if you or your husband lose your jobs? Can you really balance a full-time career and full-time motherhood? Or should you consider being a stay-at-home mom?

After some soul searching, you realize you cannot control or plan everything. The decision is made. You're going to have a baby!

Now the serious planning begins: When will I stop using birth control? When will our baby be born? How many children will we have, and when?

Don't be surprised if you feel a wave of anxiety as the first date of your "life plan" arrives and you flush the birth control pills down the toilet. As you stand on the edge of the high dive preparing to jump into the baby-making pool, you may find you have to run back to the ladder and climb down. You ask yourself, "Would it really be so bad to take a few months to enjoy our last 'free' days as a couple before we become responsible parents?" Let's call a spade a spade. You know a lot of couples with kids, and they aren't going out for sushi and a movie on a random Tuesday night. In all honesty, neither are you, but you could if you wanted to, and you vow that for the next few months you'll take full advantage of your carefree status as a kid-free couple.

Ignorance Is Bliss

Once you actually start the baby-making process, it's really fun. Multiply the fun times ten if this is your first. This becomes your favorite topic of conversation, and you and your husband spend hours talking about your life with a baby, just like the old days before marriage when you used to talk endlessly about what the rest of your life would be like together. Now when you are cornered with the "Are you trying?" gun held to your head, you no longer claim an emergency bathroom break; you just grin and slyly admit you've "pulled the goalie."

You feel closer to your husband than ever before as you move down this exciting path together. Every time you see him with a child, a surge of happiness rushes over you from head to toe. He's going to be an incredible father, and soon it will be your very own child up on his shoulders. You can't believe how exciting it all is— you're going to be a family!

Once there's no birth control in place, you may start the next level of planning: You'll turn the office into a nursery, cram the computer into your bedroom and convert the basement into an oversized playroom. More important, your newest pastime consumes you—naming your soon-to-arrive baby. Each day you find yourself offering a new suggestion to your husband. "What about Kate?" you ask. "No, I dated a girl named Kate in college," your husband replies. "What about Madeline?" he tosses back. "No, Toys "R" Us has a huge section of Madeline dolls and games. I don't want our child to be part of a franchise." And so it goes, the name game is played night after night, and you love it!

Your sex life takes on a higher purpose too—you're not just "making love," you're "making a baby." Each night resembles a romance novel, complete with candlelit dinners, fresh flowers in the bedroom and mood lighting. You feel like a honeymooner all over again, and shaving your legs becomes a daily, no longer quarterly, event. All this romance takes effort, but it's worth it. You'll smile as you look back on these days knowing your child was conceived with love.

To:	Courtney <Courtney@conceptionchronicles.com>;
	Shelly <Shelly@conceptionchronicles.com>
From:	Patty <Patty@conceptionchronicles.com>
Subject:	**News Flash**

Well girls . . . it's official. Scott and I have decided we are ready to start a family! It's so cute; he's already talking about how we could convert the garage into a playroom and build an extension on the house. It's a bit early to start the construction . . . but I have to admit, it's fun to think about a little one running around.

I'm kind of surprised nothing has happened yet, but I guess it takes a few months for the birth control to work its way out of your system, right?

It would be great if I could have the baby in May and get the summer off.

To: Courtney <Courtney@conceptionchronicles.com>;
          Patty <Patty@conceptionchronicles.com>
From: Shelly <Shelly@conceptionchronicles.com>
Subject: **RE: News Flash**

How exciting! You'll be such a great mom. Forget the addition; you'll need a whole new wing to handle all the baby toys. May would be perfect—you can get back in shape and maybe even get a tan for once. Keep me posted.

To: Patty <Patty@conceptionchronicles.com>;
          Shelly <Shelly@conceptionchronicles.com>
From: Courtney <Courtney@conceptionchronicles.com>
Subject: **RE: RE: News Flash**

Great news! I'm so happy for you and Scott. I hope the timing works that you get your summer off, but I have to tell you, it took us almost a year.

To: Courtney <Courtney@conceptionchronicles.com>;
          Shelly <Shelly@conceptionchronicles.com>
From: Patty <Patty@conceptionchronicles.com>
Subject: **WHAT??**

A YEAR??

This Is Much Harder Than You Thought

A few months pass and you're surprised you're not pregnant. Hmmm. This is a little harder than you thought. We were raised to believe we could get pregnant if we came within three miles of the male species—with or without our pants on. In fact, getting pregnant was so easy it could happen if you accidentally swallowed a watermelon seed at a barbecue. Our whole lives we lived in constant fear that any day we would just wake up pregnant. Yes, we used birth control, but the disclaimer clearly stated in six-point font that there was a 1 percent chance of pregnancy even while taking the pill. We knew it would be us.

Sure, we wised up a little over the years, but somewhere embedded deep in our being, we believed getting pregnant would never be a problem. It was staying *not pregnant* that was the challenge, at least until we had a suitable groom on our arm. But here we were, a few months flying free with no birth control . . . and nothing! Maybe all those horror stories of "nice" girls getting pregnant were meant to dissolve in our memories once we hit adulthood. Since sex was not on the menu for our family discussions, our parents often resorted to scare tactics to drive home the concept of abstinence. By the time we became sexually active, we felt like we were playing with a loaded gun. We were more than a little caught off guard when we finally reached the point in our lives when we were trying to achieve pregnancy and nothing was happening.

Ever the optimists, we didn't panic but convinced ourselves this must be normal—surprising, but normal.

Striving to Be Average

What is normal? Come to think of it, you've never really given any thought to just how long it may take to get pregnant. Surely *you* have nothing to worry about—women are having babies well into their forties. You know this for a fact because every magazine cover proudly features the over-forty celebrity du jour with her bulging belly and well-toned arms under a headline screaming, "Forty Is the New Thirty." If they can do it, so can you!

Just the Facts

At your routine checkup, you casually ask your OB-GYN how long it takes most couples to conceive. Her answer certainly wasn't what you expected. She tells you the average couple has a *10 to 20 percent* chance of conceiving each month. WHAT? Why are you just hearing this now for the first time? You may wonder what would have happened if you married your college sweetheart and started knocking out your family before graduation? Surprisingly, the success rates for couples in their twenties is only about 20 percent for each month's attempts. It may not be nice to fool Mother Nature, but she certainly has pulled one over on us.

The 10 to 20 percent success rate keeps spinning around in your head. You had a stats class in college. Sure you got a C-, but you learned enough to know that averages are the result of extremes. Maybe these findings don't really apply to you. It's time to dig in and do a little more research.

After some initial snooping around, the first thing that jumps out at you is the medical community's definition of "infertile." They consider men and women infertile after having unprotected intercourse for one year without conceiving a child. To us the word "infertile" is much more powerful—we always thought it meant barren, sterile, no chance in hell you were ever going to have kids. Not that we always have to be right, but apparently *Webster's New World Dictionary of the American Language* agrees with us. Very simply put, *Webster's* defines infertile as "not fertile [brilliant, aren't they?]; not productive; barren."

Rather than getting hung up on linguistics, you read on and learn that more than 10 percent of all couples in their childbearing years fall into this medically defined category of infertility. That's over six million men and women. Holy shit! It just doesn't make sense—how is it Gymboree stores and Chuck E. Cheese's are popping up in every strip mall across America? Clearly, *someone* is having children.

The good news is that total infertility is rare. It may take you longer than you expect or plan, and you may have to seek the help of a doctor, but the future looks bright even for those who are forced to wear the ugly label of infertile—90 percent will achieve pregnancy with treatment. These details are definitely worth discussing over dinner tonight with your husband.

It Takes Two, Baby

Husbands

The first thing you must realize as you begin your baby-making adventure is that the odds of you and your husband being on the same page emotionally are as likely as spotting Elvis at the corner deli. The sooner you accept this fact, the smoother the road will be for both of you.

The difference in your attitudes may begin to surface after a few months of failed efforts. While your husband is thanking God for his rock star sex life, you are praying to God to please make you a mother. While you view each month as a chance for motherhood, we find that most men, particularly in the beginning, view ovulation as a free pass to unlimited sex. Courtney's husband, Dan, blatantly started working it into his foreplay routine—"Are you ovulating?" along with a wink, wink. Needless to say, Courtney didn't find this the least bit romantic, but if she was indeed ovulating, she would play along. If she wasn't, she responded more honestly with something like, "No, you moron," in hopes of dissuading him from using her bodily functions as a means of seduction.

Once you begin your fertility fact-finding mission, the emotional gap may become even more evident. You think it is perfectly appropriate to start a conversation with the phrase, "Did you know . . . ?" followed by a dissertation on the odds of conceiving that month under a full moon. At this point, your husband is still trying to be supportive, so he may pretend to be listening as he asks for another serving of mashed potatoes. We guarantee if he was given a number two pencil and sent to the living room to complete an essay on your recent findings, he'd be back at the table begging for a multiple-choice alternative.

As you present each month's fast facts and new strategies for conception, the more direct husband may insist you are thinking about this pregnancy stuff way too much. He may smile as you deliver new, roomier boxers, but what he's really thinking is all you need to do is have more sex, and you'll be pregnant in no time. He takes on the cable network approach—all sex, all the time—while you remain committed to proven medical research to increase your odds.

We don't know if men are really this clueless (and please excuse us if you have the one husband on the planet who is actively charting your menstrual cycle) or if this is all part of a well-developed plot to have a killer sex life. Either way, your husband's laid-back attitude means only one thing—you are clearly going to be the alpha dog in the quest for parenthood.

Mother Knows Best

Much like the stock market, your mother's behavior can be very erratic. When dealing with the subject of procreation, the level of unpredictability may be downright shocking. If you're like us, odds are you haven't been detailing the events of your married sex life with your mother. And, it may be a long shot, but we're guessing your mother is thankful for that.

But when your efforts in the bedroom shift from pleasure to purpose, you may be very tempted to let your mother in on the exciting news. You know nothing would make her happier than becoming a grandmother, and you want her to be a part of the excitement right from the very beginning.

Even though she will undoubtedly be overjoyed by the fact you are trying to have a baby, she may not react the way you expect. Your good news may actually bring out an unattractive side of her. She's been waiting a long time to become a grandmother, and for years she's been listening to endless stories about her friends' grandchildren. It's payback time. Unless she is placed under strict house rules, she'll be on the phone to Aunt Kitty in a flash detailing your bedroom activity and bragging about her yet-to-be conceived grandchild.

Although there is no documentation to prove this, we are convinced the expression "too much information" was born from a conversation between a woman actively trying to have a baby and her supportive mother. Keep this in mind as you bring your mother into the loop. She may be thrilled with the closeness of your relationship and the fact that you trust her with your most personal issues. But the line separating the informed from the overinformed must be carefully navigated. Telling your mother you are trying to have a baby. Acceptable. Detailing the number of days in your typical menstrual cycle. Acceptable. Reviewing sexual positions that deliver maximum penetration. Unacceptable! (At least with our mothers.)

There is, however, a gray area between the clearly acceptable and unacceptable. This is where the unpredictable behavior comes into play. You'll have to gauge this for yourself, but when you start getting into the details of your and your husband's bodily functions, enter at your own risk.

In fairness to your mother, you must know that you are catching her off guard. In all of your mother's fantasies about the day she would learn she was going to be a grandmother, not one of them included a pre-grandma conversation with you about your sex life. If you are so bold to bring up your fickle ovaries and your stretchy cervical fluid, know that this is comparable to opening a vibrator at your bridal shower. Be prepared for awkward silence or nervous laughter.

We're not saying you shouldn't let your mom in on your baby-making progress. We're just letting you know from our own experiences that starting a family today, with all the tools, tests and techniques, is very different from how it was when your mother started her family. So cut your mom some slack if she doesn't react exactly like you expect when you invite her into the brave new world of baby making.

We personally have found our mothers to be incredibly supportive throughout the whole family-building ordeal. Sure, we had a few funny phone conversations, and we felt like we were teaching sex-ed at AARP at times, but at the end of the day, our mothers didn't let us down . . . and neither will yours.

Dads Don't Want to Know

Don't be hurt if your dad is especially uncomfortable or disinterested in the events leading up to the actual pregnancy. He is begging to be left in the dark. Think of your quest to get pregnant like a night for your dad at a fabulous five-star restaurant. Like everyone else, your dad probably loves to be served by an impeccably dressed waitstaff who present mouth-watering entrees and vegetables you can't pronounce.

What your dad doesn't need to know is what happened leading

up to the gourmet goodies arriving at the table. Minutes before walking out of the kitchen, the waiter dropped your father's NY Strip on the floor. Rather than holding up the order and heading back to the prep area, the waiter just brushed it off with a grimy rag, redrizzled the béarnaise and put it right back on the plate. Does your father need to know? Absolutely not. Ignorance is bliss.

And so may be the case with your pregnancy. Your parents may not be interested in what's happening behind the closed doors in the bedroom, but know for a fact they are silently supporting you. When the day finally arrives when you announce you are going to have a baby, the unbridled excitement will far outweigh the joy of, say, the Berlin Wall falling or man's first walk on the moon. If you happen to be the first daughter pregnant or if you are carrying the first grandchild, realize you are now capable of walking on water (at least in your parents' eyes).

It's Not Nice to Fool Mother Nature

After a few months of failed efforts, you start to question the necessity of having taken birth control pills for the past ten years. Birth control pills basically work by tricking your body into thinking it's already pregnant. At this rate, maybe your body is just tired from being "virtually" knocked up for the past decade. It's time you have a talk with your inner self, come clean, wake up the old ovaries and get going.

At your next OB-GYN appointment, you mention you've been trying to get pregnant but haven't had any luck yet. "Are you ovulating?" the doctor asks. After a moment of hesitation you start to mumble and then muster up a less-than-convincing "I think so." In all honesty, you really don't know if you are ovulating. You've had regular periods since the eighth grade, uneventful pap smears and an "Everything looks great" at every annual exam. You took this to assume that yes, you must be ovulating. But as far as hard-core medical proof that an egg popped out of an ovary, that's something you just don't know.

After a few more questions from your doctor about how long you've been trying (it's only been a few months) and when you're having sex (all the time), your doctor casually mentions you may want to use an ovulation kit just to be sure, but she also says, "Just keep having sex from days ten to fifteen, and you should be fine."

You weren't all that concerned before, and you're relieved to see your doctor doesn't really seem all that concerned either. But you take her advice to heart and think that yes, it is time to start monitoring your ovulation a little more closely just to make sure all the equipment is working properly.

Pinpointing your ovulation may take some of the pressure off you. Once you get a little more familiar with your cycle, you won't have to be a sex goddess twenty-four hours a day, seven days a week. Maybe now you can be a sex goddess when you're ovulating and just the plain old regular goddess the rest of the month.

chapter two

Finding Your Fertile Self

Wednesday

Notes

Thursday

Notes

- Grocery Store
- Milk
- Eggs
- Decaf
- Bananas
- Ovulation sticks

Friday

Notes

- Upgrade to high-speed Internet

If you're one of those women so in tune with your body that you can pinpoint the exact moment of your ovulation because you feel a slight twinge in your ovary, then please skip directly to chapter 3. But if you're like the rest of us—that is, you have a basic understanding of where your ovaries are, but you certainly can't distinguish between an acute appendicitis and ovarian pain—then this chapter is for you. Who knows, your body may be sending subtle messages, and you've just dismissed it as gas!

After the recent conversation with your doctor, you realize there may be a thing or two you need to learn about your body and the complicated process of conception. It's time to switch to information-gathering mode.

As embarrassing as it is to admit, when we first started trying to get pregnant, not one of us knew when we ovulated. Sure, we knew it was sometime in the middle of our cycles, but since we had been actively trying NOT to have a baby for so many years, we just assumed the minute we stopped using protection, we'd be pregnant in no time. This may work for some women, but that certainly wasn't the case for any of us. We needed to do a little research and flash back to our Biology 101 lessons on human reproduction.

So where should you start? Even though most Internet searches even remotely related to the topic of sex end up at a porn site, the World Wide Web is a logical first step.

Ready, Set, GOogle

Thank God for Google . . . the greatest search engine of all time! No more Dewey decimal system. All the information is just a click away. Up until the quest to have a baby began to take over our lives, we used Google for such noble pursuits as tracking down every guy we'd ever dated since tenth grade. If we could dig up our college boyfriend and learn he ran a 5K race in under thirty minutes in

Central Park, we certainly could learn a thing or two about the ever-elusive ovulation cycle.

Our first word of advice—please conduct your Internet searches at home or after hours at the office. Even the most harmless, scientific Web sites will undoubtedly have huge graphics of rattles, babies and loving couples embracing. If someone happens to drop by your office unexpectedly, your personal life will not be personal for long.

To: Courtney <Courtney@conceptionchronicles.com>;
           Shelly <Shelly@conceptionchronicles.com>
From: Patty <Patty@conceptionchronicles.com>
Subject: **Branded Infertile—Yikes**

You aren't going to believe what just happened. This morning I went on an ovulatory fact-finding mission at work. I logged on to Amazon and bought a few books to help me get in touch with my fertile self.

Now, whenever I log on, all of the recommended books scream INFERTILITY! Yikes! This isn't even my computer—I'm just a consultant! The computer may as well take over the intercom system and announce my arrival each day with "Good Morning, Infertile Woman."

In an attempt to throw off Big Brother, I bought a few cookbooks. No good. For some reason, my "recommended reading" list still has all the fertility books with HUGE pictures at the top, and there are only two cookbooks listed in small print on the bottom. I'm so humiliated! I have to call the help desk to get me out of this mess! HELP!

To: Patty<Patty@conceptionchronicles.com>
From: Shelly<Shelly@conceptionchronicles.com>
Cc: Courtney<Courtney@conceptionchronicles.com>
Subject: **Look before you link**

Never do a search and then start randomly cruising the fertility Web sites while you're at work. I did a search once on "conception" and just kept jumping from site to site. Of course, I landed on a few porn sites but didn't think anything of it. For months, I had a constant flow of pop-up ads declaring, "67% of women are dissatisfied with the size of their partner's penis." Poor Bruce. Luckily, he didn't develop a complex.

Gridlock on the Information Highway

You'll feel much better about your ignorance once you type the word "ovulation" into the search bar and hit Enter. We were completely shocked to find over 700,000 matching sites. Clearly, we're not the only women who have no idea when they ovulate. There is good and bad news about having so many choices to browse on the Web. The good news is there's a lot of great information to help you learn about your body and move you closer to achieving your goal of conception. The bad news is anyone who can type three *ws* in a row can put up a Web site and call themselves an expert, so you really need to sort through what's fact and what's fiction.

Here are just a few of the Web sites we liked and found to be quite helpful:

- **www.babycenter.com:** This is the go-to site for everything baby. Plus there are great chat rooms and bulletin board postings for everyone in every situation.
- **www.gettingpregnant.co.uk.:** If you like Hugh Grant, bangers and mash and the Royal Family, you'll love this Web site for beginners. It has all the basics you need to know along with a side of British wit.
- **www.iVillage.com:** This Web site for women contains many articles on pregnancy and fertility.

Don't be intimidated by the word "infertility" found on the following Web sites. Regardless of where you are in the process, these are great sites that can offer support and answer all types of questions related to fertility:

- **www.resolve.org:** The official Web site for RESOLVE: The National Infertility Association is great for information, resources and support. It also has bulletin boards categorized by where you are in the treatment process—getting started, general information and pregnancy after infertility.
- **www.ivfconnections.com:** This site is obviously for those who are seeking fertility treatment, but even those not going through IVF will find interesting information. It also hosts a series of bulletin boards broken out by age, lifestyle, diagnosis and so on.
- **www.asrm.org:** American Society for Reproductive Medicine is dedicated to infertility and reproductive medical issues. This is a good site for hard-core facts and figures.
- **www.theafa.org:** The site for the American Fertility Association offers support and provides answers to the many questions related to infertility. It also features monthly online seminars related to the topic.

Introduction to Chat Room Chatter 101

If you happen to stumble into a chat room or try to read some of the bulletin board postings on these sites, you will probably feel like the only nonsorority sister at Greek Week. The acronyms fly free in these chat fests. We managed to decipher a few of them on our own, but many left us scratching our heads in utter confusion. To save you the trouble, here's a little fertility chat room cheat sheet:

Chat Room Lingo for Beginners

2ww	Two week wait after ovulation
AF	Aunt Flo (flow), in other words, your period
AI	Artificial Insemination
AO	Anovulation
ART	Assisted Reproductive Technology
ASA	Anti-Sperm Antibody
BB	Bulletin Board
BBT	Basal Body Temperature
BCP	Birth Control Pills
BD	Baby Dancing (sex)
BFN	Big Fat Negative (pregnancy test result)
BFP	Big Fat Positive (pregnancy test result)
BMS	Baby-Making Sex
B/W	Bloodwork
CD	Cycle Day
CM	Cervical Mucus
DE	Donor Eggs
DI	Donor Insemination
DPO	Days Post-Ovulation
DPR	Days Post-Retrieval (IVF)
DPT	Days Post-Transfer (IVF)
DP3DT	Days Post 3-Day Transfer
DP5DT	Days Post 5-Day Transfer
Dx	Diagnosis
E2	Estradiol (Estrogen)
EPT	Early Pregnancy Test
ET	Embryo Transfer (IVF)
FET	Frozen Embryo Transfer
FSH	Follicle Stimulating Hormone
FV	Fertile Vibes
HPT	Home Pregnancy Test

IF	Infertility
IUI	Intrauterine Insemination
IVF	In Vitro Fertilization
LAP	Laparoscopy
LH	Luteinizing Hormone
LP	Luteal Phase
LPD	Luteal Phase Defect
MC, m/c	Miscarriage
O, OV	Ovulation
OPT	Ovulation Predictor Test
OTC	Over the Counter
PCOS	Polycystic Ovary Syndrome
PCT	Postcoital Test
PG	Pregnant
PI	Primary Infertility
RE	Reproductive Endocrinologist
SA	Semen Analysis
SI	Secondary Infertility
TMI	Too Much Information
TTC	Trying To Conceive
UR	Urologist
US, u/s	Ultrasound

In addition to the basic medical terms just listed above, there is also a secret code for members of the family:

DD Darling Daughter
DH Darling Husband
DS Darling Son
DW Darling Wife
MIL Mother-in-Law (FIL, BIL, SIL for the other in-laws)

Interesting point to note: everyone in the family is "darling" except the in-laws. Clearly, whoever masterminded these abbreviations had issues. When we first logged on to these bulletin boards, we immediately assumed DH stood for "damn," not "darling," husband. Of course, our husbands annoy us as much as the next wife, but we were a little surprised these poor men were bombarded with constant belligerence on the boards. When we finally realized they were not being reamed so much as revered, the finger pointed right back at us. Forgive us, but the last time we heard anyone refer to her spouse as "darling" was on a *Leave It to Beaver* episode.

At first glance, these bulletin boards may come off as kind of corny. Come on, who needs an abbreviation for sex? It's only three letters, and the abbreviation, BD, is two. So what, you save one letter? We're all adults. Why can't we say, "My husband and I had sex last night," as opposed to "DH and I BD last night"?

When you're chatting on the boards and someone wants to send you good luck, they "sprinkle baby dust" or "send baby dust your way." Yes, we live in a Disney-loving society, so we're assuming sprinkling baby dust is intended to get us pregnant much like Tinkerbell's sprinkling of fairy dust allowed Peter Pan to fly. This was a little too much for us, so we opted for the old-fashioned "good luck" for our online well wishes.

Once you get past the corniness of the chat room lingo, these bulletin boards can be an incredible source of information and support. There should be a warning attached that once you post, you are in danger of becoming instantly addicted. Having never been in a chat room or posted on a bulletin board prior to the fertility sites, we were amazed at how quickly you become invested in other people's lives and how much support people in a similar situation can provide that others cannot—not to mention the benefit of having a checks-and-balance system over your medical care provider's advice and treatment. With the click of a button, you have hundreds of women, along with their experience, to ask questions, confirm diagnoses and review treatment recommendations. So grab your chat room cheat sheet and log on.

What's on Your Nightstand?

Since you're holding this book in your hand, you've probably already started to explore the many books available on fertility. We bought countless books on what to eat, how to exercise and what to wear (i.e., no tighty whities for the mister). We were both relieved and overwhelmed when we made the first trips to bookstores and found literally hundreds of titles promising us motherhood. There are entire books dedicated to subjects like acupuncture, which we had not even considered at this point—but more on that later. The fact is, if you are interested in a particular topic as it relates to fertility, the information is out there; you just need to find it.

The one book we strongly recommend to everyone trying to conceive is Toni Weschler's *Taking Charge of Your Fertility*. This book is the encyclopedia of all that is female and answers everything from the most basic questions about your menstrual cycle to the more daunting concerns around assisted reproductive technology. The book is easy to read and packed full of information. In particular, Ms. Weschler teaches us how to interpret our bodies' natural signs, which alert us to our pending ovulation through temperature and cervical fluid changes.

Knowledge is power, so polish up that credit card and fill your bookshelf with as many books on fertility as you can devour. But before you make yourself crazy with all-night read-a-thons, remember, these books are merely tools to help you. Pick and choose the information that works best for you, and toss aside the other 3 million recommendations you uncover along the way.

The Friends and Family Plan

As you begin your search for information on pregnancy, your most natural urge will be to pick up the phone and call every mother you know. Before you do, we have one thing to say—don't! Starting a dialogue on conception is basically synonymous with taking out a full-page ad in *The New York Times*. Remember the Breck shampoo commercial from the 1970s . . . and they told two friends, and so on and so on? If you think people like talking about a great shampoo, imagine the field day they'll have with your baby-making efforts.

Of course, we're not suggesting you lock yourself away in an isolation booth until you're wearing the latest designs from Mimi Maternity. We're merely recommending you put a little thought into your circle of fertility friends before you take advantage of your flat-rate calling plan.

We divided our friends into three distinct groups: the inner, the fringe and the outer. First, there's the inner circle of friends. This small group was fully in the know of every gory detail—daily temperature, sexual activity and each month's results. These were our closest friends who had either been through a prolonged baby-making process, so there was no need for an explanation when you dropped a bombshell about your latest sexual encounter, or were the type of friends who offer unwavering support even though they haven't been through the same ordeal themselves.

Next, there are the fringe friends. Rather than basking in the hot sun of every detail like the inner circle, this group is kept in the shade. Yes, they may know you are trying to get pregnant, but no, they don't know you have a doctor's appointment on Wednesday at 10 A.M. to inspect your ovaries. This lack of information doesn't make this group any less of a friend than the inner circle; however, you may choose to spare the fringe friends from the minutiae.

And finally the outer circle. We struggled with not telling these friends about our plans to get pregnant, especially when they asked. But for any number of reasons, you may decide it's best to keep some of your friends in the dark about your efforts in the bedroom. Most of our single girlfriends fell into this category. While they're battling the minefields of dating, why should we burden them with a sneak preview of the potential challenges of achieving pregnancy? Friendships are not built on one common interest, so focus on the many other activities that brought you together as friends in the first place. Believe it or not, these friends will become a great source of relief the longer it takes to become pregnant. You can be sure a night out with the outer circle will not start with the dreaded question, "Any news?" and the conversation at dinner will thankfully revolve around politics and the latest shopping bargains rather than pregnancy and the sleeping patterns of a two-month-old.

For those of you who are open books and love to share every detail of your personal lives with the world, by all means scream from the rooftop that you are having unprotected sex. But for everyone else, hold your tongue. We know you are anxious to share the excitement with your friends and family—so were we. Until you are actually pregnant, however, you have no idea how long it's going to take or what you're going to have to go through to get there, so it might be wise to hold your cards a little close. If you're lucky, you'll be pregnant in no time, and all your friends will move directly to the inner circle and endure countless hours of hearing every detail of your pregnancy.

The Big "O"—It's Not Just for Orgasm Anymore

No wonder you're not pregnant yet—you had no idea what you were doing. But now that you've spent countless hours on the Internet, at the bookstore and chatting with your inner circle of friends, you are on full fertility alert.

Once we knew our cervical fluid would take on a stretchy, egg-white quality as we approached our fertile windows, our trips to the restroom had little to do with relieving our bladders. One book Patty read actually said, "Be aware of your vagina throughout your cycle." Patty could honestly say she had neglected her vagina up until that point; but once she was aware of the daily changes happening in her body, her vagina became a top priority.

In addition to the increase of slimy cervical fluid, some women actually feel a cramp right around the time they ovulate. This pain is called *mittelschmerz*, which means "midcycle pain." Say this to a doctor, and you will most certainly impress. Say this in a deli, and you will end up with cream cheese on your bagel. We were never lucky enough to experience *mittelschmerz*, or any *schmerz* for that matter, but we know TTCs who swore they felt the twinge, hit the sack and nine months later their bundle of joy arrived.

There are many reasons why your attempts to procreate fail, but at the end of the day, it comes down to all the planets aligning. Everything needs to be just right in your body—the hormones, the cervical fluid, the egg, the fallopian tubes, the cervical lining. And then, everything needs to be just right in your husband's body—he needs to have enough sperm with enough motivation to make the journey and find its golden egg.

Fertility Fables

When you talk to your girlfriends in the inner circle, each will undoubtedly have her own advice on what you should do to overcome your fertility challenges. Some of these tidbits of wisdom may have come from their own experiences, while others may be a third-party referral from their Aunt Betty's cousin Martha's sister Sally. Needless to say, this advice may not be based on any hardcore medical findings, and we do not recommend pinning your hopes for children on them. Nevertheless, here are a few of our favorites that left us speechless.

1. *Check the color of your vulva.* This is something only your closest friend would suggest. We can't remember the last time we used the word "vulva" in a sentence, especially when doling out advice to others. But one of our TTCs swore that her "lips" took on a purple color when she ovulated. We're not even going to ask how she discovered this—clearly she was in touch with her feminine side. We were just grateful to finally have a use for the multitude of minimirrors we've received over the years as free gifts with our cosmetic purchases.

2. *Watch for rectal spasms.* Apparently some women notice spasms in their rectum as they approach ovulation. It goes without saying, these women clearly have too much time on their hands if they are keeping track of what any normal human being would assume was a bean burrito acting up. We never followed up on this advice other than to send each other funny e-mails about our spastic rectums.

3. *Inject egg whites into your vagina.* Cervical fluid is crucial for the

sperm to successfully make the journey from its drop-off point through the cervix into the fallopian tube to eventually meet up with the egg. If you don't have enough cervical fluid, the sperm stop dead in their tracks. So another of our TTCs told us we could inject egg whites into our vaginas before having sex, which would act as a substitute for the missing-in-action cervical fluid. We're not certain, but this probably doesn't count toward your daily protein intake if you're following the Atkins Diet. Our TTC swore she read this in *Taking Charge of Your Fertility.* We were skeptical at first, but we did actually find it in the book, along with a warning you could possibly contract salmonella by using eggs in this way. We say better safe than sorry—for now, why not just keep your eggs in the frying pan?

Bag of Ovulation Tricks

You may feel like you've just earned your Ph.D. in human reproduction—that's certainly the way we felt! However, if all of this new knowledge still has not brought about results, why not stack the deck in your favor and move on to the abundance of fertility-tracking paraphernalia available to you. There are plenty of tools that will help identify your fertile days and should increase your chances of getting pregnant. Little did we know when we opened up the ovulation toolbox, the infamous "forty-eight fertile hours" would soon turn into ten anxiety-laden days.

We each tried a combination of do-it-yourself tests and found varying and limited degrees of success. Unfortunately, these kits and tools can't be purchased with your corporate flexible spending account, so brace yourself—it could get expensive!

Ovulation Predictor Kits—Warning: May Not Be for Everyone

What could be easier than peeing on a stick? The ovulation predictor kits are one of the quickest ways to zero in on your peak fertile days. The sticks come seven to a box, which clearly is not enough for the TTC "heavy user." We're not sure if the manufacturers were trying to be optimistic, or if we just overindulged. Either way, our advice is to double up on your maiden purchase—one box is never enough.

The instructions suggest you begin testing (aka peeing on the stick) around day nine, depending on the number of days in your cycle. Expect ovulation twenty-four to thirty-six hours after you see a solid blue line that matches the test line of the ovulation stick. This line indicates the luteinizing hormone (LH) surge in your urine and lets you know an egg is going to be released. Sound simple enough? Well, it's not. Van Gogh would have difficulty interpreting the shades of blue hues found on an ovulation stick. After a particularly frustrating month, Shelly found herself digging through her husband's toolbox in search of his high-power flashlight to verify the unreadable results in her dimly lit bathroom. If the line almost matched, did that mean she was almost ovulating?

The downside to the ovulation sticks, and their not-quite-clear results, is they often lead to obsessive behavior. Shelly convinced herself she was missing her ovulation window and began testing twice a day, on day five. This is not recommended! You will waste a ton of money and drive yourself insane. Admitting you have a problem is the first step. Once Shelly took a look at the trash can full of discarded wrappers, she realized this may not be the best tool for her. It was time for an upgrade to the fertility monitor.

Fertility Monitor—The "Uber" Stick

If you can force yourself to read and reread the instruction manual for the fertility monitor, you will save yourself a major headache. And so it begins. You're still peeing on sticks, but this time an electronic monitor will be leading the ovulation charge. Based on the day of your cycle, the monitor will inform you if a test stick is required that day. After receiving your prompt, you have exactly fifteen seconds to pee on the stick and insert it properly into the monitor for an accurate reading. If in your haste you (a) insert the stick incorrectly, (b) get the monitor wet, (c) don't pee on the stick long enough or (d) any number of other unforgivable errors, the monitor will definitely let you know by flashing a bold exclamation point! It might as well scream, "You idiot!" If this all sounds demanding and intimidating, rest assured, it is.

This new tool is loaded with visuals, like the picture of an egg ready to burst free and a bar graph indicating your low, medium and high fertile days. For some, it can be an overwhelming way to track your fertility. For us, it was a way to conduct our own scientific experiment by simultaneously using the ovulation predictor sticks and the fertility monitor to check for inconsistencies. All that was missing was a white lab coat, goggles and a high-powered microscope. If you find yourself in this predicament, STOP. You've gone too far. You are in ovulation overload.

From Russia with Love—The Spitnik (aka Ovulite™)

If you find you have an unpredictable cycle, the Ovulite may be for you. Little did we know that Courtney was on the cutting edge of fertility tracking devices with her Russian ovulation predictor tool. Her doctor recommended this high-tech device from Russia (we've affectionately named it the *Spitnik*) because her cycles were so unpredictable it was impossible to rely on the ovulation predictor sticks alone.

At the time, the Spitnik did not have FDA approval for distribution in the United States, but her doctor was so convinced of its merits, he imported his own supply and kept a private stash in his credenza. After a brief explanation in the doctor's office, which went in one ear and out the other, Courtney was left to her own devices to decipher the Russian instructions.

Essentially, the Spitnik is a lipstick-shaped minimicroscope that can be discreetly tucked away in any purse. Each day, you put a drop of saliva on the piece of glass and then examine it through the spylike microscope. If you see spots and lines, you are not fertile. If you see a fern pattern among the spots and lines, you will probably ovulate in three to four days. If you see a full fern pattern, your egg is itching to pop out at any minute.

In Courtney's case, it was a two-part predictor process—Spitnik fern patterns confirmed possible ovulation, which meant it was time to pee on the stick and, hopefully, see blue lines. The combination worked wonders. The only hitch was Courtney needing to radio her husband back from a business trip—a small price to pay when you've reached your fertile window. It's been said, "Hell hath no fury like a woman scorned." Our husbands would disagree; it should rather be, "Hell hath no fury like a woman ovulating!"

Luckily for you, the days of underground Spitnik distribution are over. The FDA has approved the tool for use in the United States, and it is now available for sale under the name Ovulite. More good news, the directions are in English, so no need to learn a second language.

Temperature Charting—Six Degrees of Separation

We always thought of the natural family-planning method as something the Mormons used; based on the size of their families, we never even considered it as a method of birth control. But once the shoe was on the other foot, we thought any method that was so ineffective at preventing pregnancy surely must be effective in helping to achieve it. On the recommendation of a TTC, Patty set out on a "natural" course to become one with her body.

After digging through her medicine cabinet, Patty realized her old-fashioned mercury thermometer wouldn't cut it for the job of monitoring her slight body temperature variations. After purchasing two different types of digital thermometers, she finally got it right when she bought the basal body temperature thermometer. If you're having a hard time finding the right thermometer, just look for the one with the huge baby and promises of pregnancy on the box.

Unless you keep a stash of graph paper on hand, we recommend buying the computer program *Taking Charge of Your Fertility*, based on the book of the same name by Toni Weschler. Basically, you take your temperature first thing in the morning, at approximately the same time each day. Then you log your results into the program, and a diagnosis is made: not fertile, low fertility, high fertility, ovulation, post ovulation. The trick here is that literally the only movement you're allowed before taking your temperature is a slow-motion roll over to the side of the bed, grabbing the thermometer and popping it in your mouth. When your temperature spikes, it means you've ovulated. Unfortunately, it takes a couple of cycles before the computer can predict your most fertile days.

Many of our TTCs swear by this method, but Patty found it to be a bit annoying. Not being a morning person, half the time she would be on her way to the bathroom before she realized she forgot to take her temperature, and another day would be lost. So if you're someone who wakes up fresh, clear-minded and ready to face the day, by all means give this a try. If you're someone who needs to be dragged out of bed and can barely function before your morning coffee, you may want to consider one of the many other tools available.

Other Tools to Consider—Online Ovulation Help

Not only can you calculate your mortgage payments online, but now finding your peak fertile days is a mouse click away. Many of the fertility-related Web sites offer ovulation predictor calculators. Just plug in your last menstrual cycle, the number of days in your cycle and voilà—your expected ovulation date. What could be easier?

We were a bit skeptical when we first tried the ovulation predictor calculators, but we found if your cycle is very consistent, they are surprisingly accurate. We wouldn't recommend using this as your only ovulation tool, but it comes in handy if you need to plan a trip to the in-laws. You'll be a little more aggressive securing the private room and letting everyone else fight about who's going to sleep on the foldout couch.

To: Patty <Patty@conceptionchronicles.com>
From: Shelly <Shelly@conceptionchronicles.com>
Cc: Courtney <Courtney@conceptionchronicles.com>
Subject: **Get on the stick**

If you haven't already tried the ovulation predictor sticks, they're amazing. It's the easiest way to really know when you're ovulating. A little advice, buy more than one box, they're definitely addictive.

To: Patty <Patty@conceptionchronicles.com>
From: Courtney <Courtney@conceptionchronicles.com>
Cc: Shelly <Shelly@conceptionchronicles.com>
Subject: **RE: Get on the stick**

I agree with Shelly, the sticks are great IF you have a regular cycle. Unfortunately, my cycle was really wacky. I would go 40–50 days in between periods. I had no clue when I ovulated, so I preferred the Spitnik. You may want to try it. I swear it's the only reason I got pregnant.

To:	Courtney <Courtney@conceptionchronicles.com>;
	Shelly <Shelly@conceptionchronicles.com>
From:	Patty <Patty@conceptionchronicles.com>
Subject:	**RE: RE: Get on the stick**

I'm already a stick addict. If I had unlimited funds, I would literally test myself every day of the month. Haven't heard anything about the Spitnik, but I think I'm good with the sticks for now.

You Are What You Eat

Once starting the conception process, many women move into the "my body is a temple" mode. If you take great joy in whipping up fresh carrot juice for breakfast, then more power to you. We had ourselves so worked up from all the information about how diet affects fertility, we were terrified to go near a cup of coffee or a glass of wine. Before you make yourself crazy with the half-caff, no-caff choice, talk to your doctor. Sure, we understood this was probably not the time to be doing shots of tequila, but wouldn't the population growth in Italy come to a complete halt if an occasional glass of wine lead to sterility? What's frustrating is there's so much information available, but much of it is conflicting. Along with doing some research, we talked with our doctors to try to answer the many questions about what we should eat, how we should exercise and how we should watch our weight. Their answer? Unless you are excessively overweight or underweight, moderation should be your guideline.

I'll Have the Number Two Platter

We all struggle when it comes to proper nutrition. It's pretty basic really—you know the foods you should and should not eat. Doctors will tell you that eating from the five food groups is essential in providing yourself with proper nutrition. But it's a lot easier said than done. However, a few small changes can go a long way. If you're having a bowl of cereal for breakfast, pass on the sugary ones offering temporary tattoos and free movie tickets. Instead, choose something more "grown-up" and throw in a sliced banana. Regardless of what's on the menu for dinner, toss in a few extra vegetables. Before you know it, you'll be at your daily requirement. And be certain to take a prenatal vitamin with the recommended daily dosage of folic acid, which aids in the prevention of birth defects.

Do You Consider a Jogging Suit Daywear?

We all know exercise is good for us. Even so, you either love it or you don't. If you're an avid exerciser, your doctor will applaud your efforts but will most likely tell you to shelve your plans to run the Boston Marathon. If you are one of those women who consider walking out to get your mail exercise, we need to talk. The next time you head to the mailbox to get your weekly dose of celebrity gossip from *People* magazine, just keep going and circle the block. If you find yourself feeling claustrophobic jamming into an elevator with ten other people, take the stairs. You'll be surprised what a brisk walk and a little exercise a few times a week will do for your mental and physical health.

To: Courtney <Courtney@conceptionchronicles.com>;
           Shelly <Shelly@conceptionchronicles.com>
From: Patty <Patty@conceptionchronicles.com>
Subject: **Turning over a new leaf**

Last night I went to the gym for a power step class. I decided I should start my new health routine now and lose a few pounds before I get pregnant.

Based on my attendance record at the gym, the 60-minute step class (which was only 55 minutes for me because I pretended I had to tie my shoe during the brutal lunges) cost me $300 bucks. That's about $5/minute!

P.S. On my way home, I ate a sloppy joe and a brownie as a last indulgence before I get crazy with the "my body is a temple" mode.

To: Patty <Patty@conceptionchronicles.com>;
           Shelly <Shelly@conceptionchronicles.com>
From: Courtney <Courtney@conceptionchronicles.com>
Subject: **RE: Turning over a new leaf**

If you're going to skip the lunges, you should probably skip the brownie, too.

When Average Is Good Enough

When it comes to weight, don't forget the Goldilocks theory—no pregnancy for you if you are too fat or too thin. You need to be *just* right. If you've grown accustomed to skipping meals and heading for the size 2 clothing rack or indulging in the coffee room jelly donuts every day, you may want to reconsider your eating habits. The bottom line is, maintaining a healthy weight is important whether or not you are trying to conceive. Talk to your doctor to be certain you fall within an acceptable weight range.

Café, Coffee, Cappuccino, Latte, Café au Lait, Cup of Joe

Is there anyone out there who doesn't drink coffee? How can we possibly help ourselves when we pass five Starbucks on the way to the office? When you're trying to get pregnant, coffee is the "wild card." While most doctors will not insist you stop all caffeine consumption, most will recommend you limit your coffee intake to two cups a day. Don't forget that caffeine is also found in such indulgent treats as chocolate, tea and regular and diet soda, so plan your snacks accordingly.

The Weekend Factor

We're fairly certain most of your evenings don't include tossing back several double vodka martinis, but it's worth a mention. Research shows excessive alcohol consumption can impair fertility. Use common sense and moderation. When we talked to our doctors, they assured us that while trying to conceive, a glass of wine with dinner is fine.

The one vice every doctor will agree is out of the question is cigarette smoking. If you're a smoker, it's time to stop (and that includes the wacky weed). A note for hubby: smoking marijuana has been shown to impair a man's fertility.

Natural Doesn't Necessarily Mean Good for You

The verdict is out on natural herbs when you're trying to get pregnant. Although you may think you are helping yourself when switching from a double espresso to an herbal tea, some of the teas may contain ingredients that interfere with pregnancy. Our advice is to stay away from all herbal supplements until you consult with your doctor.

When we finally asked our doctor about all these "rules," we were pleasantly surprised at her attitude. Her advice was, "Everything in moderation." If you look forward to a cup of coffee in the morning, go ahead and have one, but make it one, not five cups throughout the day. A glass of wine at dinner is fine—it's not a good idea to pop the cork and slug back the whole bottle, but a lovely glass of chardonnay may be the perfect answer to a long stressful day. So take this advice for what it's worth, but remember to talk to your doctor first. If you're like us, you're not going to relax about these issues until you've heard it directly from a medical professional.

Who Knew?

By now, you realize there's a lot more that goes into this whole pregnancy process than a few candles and a nice dinner followed by a romp in the hay. It may take a little longer, and you may need to use a few extra tools to get there. But at the end of the day, it's the results that matter.

So break out your sticks, thermometers and monitors—you have work to do!

chapter three

If the Stick Is Blue, You Know What to Do!

Saturday	Notes
	- *Ovulating! Must have sex!*

Sunday	Notes	Monday	Notes
	- *Must have sex!*		- *Must have sex!*

Check, Please!

When you first started down the baby-making road, you were in a dead sprint and filled with optimism. Not realizing you were getting a bit ahead of yourself, you started making elaborate plans as to how you would announce your husband's pending fatherhood. Trips to the mall included a special detour to check out the latest maternity fashions, and you secretly started making a list of the must-have items for spring for those sporting a bulging belly.

Now that you've dipped into the bag of ovulation tricks and are actively using your tool of choice but still have nothing to show for it, you are starting to feel winded. How much longer is this going to take? You flash back to ninth grade and hear the droning voice of your algebra teacher, "If you are thirty-five years old and ovulate once a month, what is the probability you will have a child by age thirty-seven?" As if that's not enough, you take your calculations to the next level to determine how quickly you'll have to get pregnant again to have your second child before you hit forty.

The frazzled frenzy of age versus fertility can leave anyone feeling a bit overwhelmed. It's time for a reality check. No, it doesn't look like you'll be one of those lucky women whose pregnancy is a "surprise," but you are also a far cry from birthing the first human clone. From all your research, you know most doctors recommend a woman consult her physician after trying to conceive for a year (if she's under thirty-five) or after six months (if she's over thirty-five). You're not there yet, so don't panic. Dust yourself off, shake off the past months' disappointments and get back to business—it's time for Operation Ovulation!

Preoperative Work: Getting the Goods

Operation Ovulation begins the minute the red flag of failure arrives. Once again, it's time for a trip to the pharmacy to pick up the monthly care package: one large box of tampons, two boxes of ovulation kits, two boxes of pregnancy tests.

In the early days of Operation Ovulation, you probably approached the checkout register rather sheepishly and tried to camouflage your conception care package by piling on all sorts of unnecessary merchandise—Pringles variety pack, every possible flavor of Twizzlers, mango body scrub and a veritable collection of celebrity rags. Buying junk food and junk journalism is probably no less embarrassing, but somehow it manages to mask the awkwardness.

Now that you are a more seasoned veteran, you have mapped out a strategy for each month. Selecting the proper retail outlet is the crucial first step. In the old days, you loved the small local pharmacy because everyone knew your name, and more than once the pharmacist questioned your choice of over-the-counter cough medicine. When it comes to Operation Ovulation, however, anonymity is key! You've scouted out the county and found one of those superstores that could double as an airport terminal with the most apathetic, disinterested, least customer-friendly pharmacy within a twenty-mile radius. Perfect!

Once all the goods are collected, it's time to check out. Not too fast! Take a moment to scan all the cashiers. You're looking for the most disgruntled (preferably male) cashier. Your ideal checker will have a dirty, rumpled uniform—a sure sign his probation officer made him take the job. Jackpot! Now just slink through the line without making eye contact or starting any small talk, and you're home free, at least for another month.

There was a month Patty was certain she was pregnant. Unfortunately, this happened almost every month, but this one month in particular she was really convinced, so she decided it was time to take a pregnancy test. She didn't have any in the house, so she ran out to the local pharmacy. Patty grabbed a pregnancy test and headed straight for the checkout line without any thought. Ironically, there was a five-foot poster declaring the store's commitment to the "Privacy Act" posted at the register. It turned out her cashier was a sweet older immigrant woman. With a thick Polish accent, she screamed, "Congratulations—Baby!" Humiliated and terrified that she may actually know someone in the long line behind her, Patty tried to explain she wasn't sure if she was pregnant, which is why she needed the test. Unfortunately, her explanation was lost in translation, and the cashier sadly replied, "You no happy with baby?" Patty didn't have the energy to explain she would be out of her mind with happiness if she were in fact pregnant, but she had been taking these tests for months and not one had been positive. Instead, she just said, "Yes, I'm very happy to be pregnant," and never went back to that store again.

Pregame Planning

Once you have purchased all the tools you need for the upcoming procreation games, it's time to get the calendar out and start planning. Don't be surprised if your attitude takes a drastic shift for the worse as the months tick by. In the beginning, we would pull out the giant wall calendar and sit down with our husbands to map out what days we thought we'd be ovulating. Then we would try to make plans for a special dinner or even a few days away at a romantic bed and breakfast during the peak days.

Unfortunately, that didn't last very long. Soon the goal of a charming B&B weekend was abandoned, and we were happy if we could manage our travel schedules long enough to be in the same state when the sneaky egg popped out. Long pregame conversations with our husbands were replaced with short, but polite, e-mails such as, "Your services will be required this month from the twenty-first until the twenth-eighth. All business trips must be preapproved by me. Have a nice day!"

Spontaneous Ovulation

Just when you take a moment to pat yourself on the back for your flawless execution leading up to O-day, the unthinkable happens . . . spontaneous ovulation. You let your guard down for only one day, and as far as you know it's too early for the stick to go off, but there it is, undeniably positive ovulation test results three days early.

How could this happen? Between the temperature charting, the ovulation sticks and the Spitnik, your body is under more intense surveillance than the White House. But you know what they say about the best-laid plans.

No matter how much preplanning you've done, or how many fertility tracking tools are currently in rotation, there are going to be months when your body exercises its prerogative to be fickle. Shelly learned this the hard way. We had planned a working weekend in Chicago to work on this book. Shelly had started trying for her second child, while Patty was deep in the throes of trying for number one. It was no small feat coordinating three schedules between ovulation cycles, business trips and personal obligations. Unexpectedly, Shelly got her period a week early and had to cancel the trip at the last minute, not wanting to risk her key fertile days away from home.

So stay focused as you inch toward your expected ovulation date. Build in a few extra days on either side, and be prepared to get home quickly if you must be out of town.

All Systems Are Go

It's hard to describe the feeling that rushes over you when your predictor stick tests positive. Whether it's the blue line on the stick or the fern pattern on the Spitnik, you feel a combination of excitement (the day you've been waiting for is finally here), hope (maybe this will be the month) and fear (it's happening right now, what if I miss it?). It is the combination of these emotions, with fear and anxiety leading the pack, that can lead to some bad bedroom behavior.

To: Shelly <Shelly@conceptionchronicles.com>;
           Courtney <Courtney@conceptionchronicles.com>
From: Patty <Patty@conceptionchronicles.com>
Subject: **The new me**

When we first started trying, I was so excited I wanted to let Scott in on every detail. The first time my ovulation stick tested positive, I was like a giggling teenager as I showed it to him and said, "If the stick is blue, you know what to do." We had a little chuckle and headed straight to the bedroom.

Fast-forward six months. There is nothing remotely cute or the least bit funny about these sticks. I'm so afraid I'm going to miss my fertile window, I'm actually testing twice a day—morning and night! Sound familiar?

When the stick finally went off last night, it was like a five-alarm fire. I actually waved it in Scott's face and yelled, "COME ON!" as I plowed past him tearing off my clothes on the way to the bedroom.

In the light of the morning, I realized my little episode could not possibly be appealing on any level, but Scott was a good sport and played along. I don't know what happened. As soon as I saw that little blue line I went crazy. Let's just hope this is the month, and I can go back to the old me.

To: Patty <Patty@conceptionchronicles.com>
From: Courtney <Courtney@conceptionchronicles.com>
Cc: Shelly <Shelly@conceptionchronicles.com>
Subject: **I feel your pain**

It feels like yesterday that I was in the same boat. Pace yourself (and your insanity). The longer it takes, the worse it gets.

To: Patty <Patty@conceptionchronicles.com>
From: Shelly <Shelly@conceptionchronicles.com>
Cc: Courtney <Courtney@conceptionchronicles.com>
Subject: **I married Keith Richards**

Patty, it's the stress that's starting to get to you. Don't beat yourself up; I'm sure Scott understands.

Bruce, on the other hand, is loving his rock star sex life since we've started trying for number two. I just got my period, and he had the gall to do his best Keith Richard's imitation and say, "When do we get back at it, babe?"

Sex on Demand

Unless you've dabbled in prostitution, the concept of sex on demand is probably foreign to you. What exactly is sex on demand? It's sex with a sole purpose—making a baby.

When your stick goes off and announces the fertile window has arrived, the bolt of energy that surges through your body is much like the startling shock you get when you plug in your blow dryer with wet hands. The only information your brain can process is "blue line + sex = baby." You know this is your only chance, and if you miss the window of opportunity, you are one month further away from motherhood.

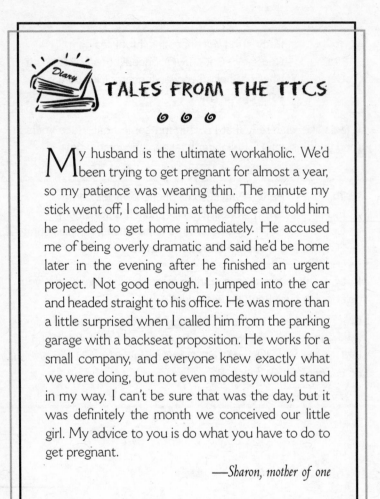

TALES FROM THE TTCS

ᕲ ᕲ ᕲ

My husband is the ultimate workaholic. We'd been trying to get pregnant for almost a year, so my patience was wearing thin. The minute my stick went off, I called him at the office and told him he needed to get home immediately. He accused me of being overly dramatic and said he'd be home later in the evening after he finished an urgent project. Not good enough. I jumped into the car and headed straight to his office. He was more than a little surprised when I called him from the parking garage with a backseat proposition. He works for a small company, and everyone knew exactly what we were doing, but not even modesty would stand in my way. I can't be sure that was the day, but it was definitely the month we conceived our little girl. My advice to you is do what you have to do to get pregnant.

—*Sharon, mother of one*

TALES FROM THE TTCS

Diary

💿 💿 💿

We had just started our baby-making efforts when we began a major construction project on our home. Between the knocked-down walls, the transparent plastic tarps functioning as doors and the team of countless contractors, privacy was scarce. Luckily, my husband was home when my stick went off, but we couldn't imagine how we could possibly work on our own expansion project. I sneaked him into the one working bathroom, locked the door and ran the shower for cover. I can only imagine what was going through the minds of the construction workers as they hammered away—"He's one lucky bastard."

—Liz, TTC

Foreplay Is for Rookies

Under normal circumstances, there is a dance of seduction that happens between most couples, which may include back massages, candlelit dinners or long intimate conversations. For most women, sexual intercourse is the big dip at the end of the tango and is the ultimate culmination of both a physical and an emotional connection with their husbands.

Sex on demand is a whole new ballgame. Your sweet flirty self may be replaced with a woman who yells, "It's time!" as a signal to begin amorous relations. All of sudden, the emotional connection that was so crucial in the past is completely disregarded. Unfortunately, ovulation sex is all about the physical result. As your husband is cozying up, you may be so bold as to tell him to skip the previews and get right to the main attraction.

While your husband may be initially attracted to the aggressive new you, the pit crew mentality, in-and-out service in less than ten minutes, may start to wear thin. You may be surprised when you start to feel a bit of reluctance from him as you call his services into action. Since when did sex have to be special for him? In your old life, your husband could have one leg caught in a bear trap and would still somehow manage to have sex if you showed even the slightest interest. Getting in the mood was an oxymoron—was there ever a time when he wasn't in the mood?

Now the roles have reversed—he is the sensitive one, and you are the one who wants sex for sex. One morning, one of our TTCs was going through her normal morning routine when she realized her test stick was sporting a bright blue line. Her husband was shaving at the sink next to her, so she immediately slammed the test stick down in front of him, with both force and urgency, and charged back to the bedroom. All this was done, as was the sex, without saying a word.

This sudden shift in the relationship is sure to leave both parties a little off balance and can have dire consequences if ignored. Try to remember how you felt when your husband would grab at you at the most insensitive times (like during your favorite reality television show). Now he's the one feeling less than loved as you hunt him down mercilessly during the mating season.

Since you have no idea how long you'll be cast in these roles, it's best to get your true feelings out in the open immediately. While you may be slightly annoyed your husband has changed the rules and now requires some level of intimacy before engaging in sex, this may not be such a bad thing. You don't want the poor guy to feel like he's only there to make a sperm donation (even if he is).

Of course, you will always feel a sense of panic when the stick turns blue, but take a deep breath and realize it's the pressure to perform that brings out the worst in you. While the goal of sex during your fertile window will always be the same, don't lose sight of some sense of romance. Would some soft music and a few candles really be so bad? You're ultimately going to end up at the same destination; why not enjoy the view along the way? Sex on demand will never be inspired by spontaneity, but that doesn't mean with a little effort and some deep breathing it can't be a meaningful experience.

A Little Effort Goes a Long Way

After a nice long talk with your husband, you realize making a baby is no time for a dictatorship. This should be a team effort, and you're happy to hear your husband wants to take a more active role in the process. You both agree that yes, you have gotten a little crazy in the past, and yes, you are both willing to make more effort so sex on demand, although planned, is actually enjoyable for both of you.

While you're beating yourself up over your previous bad boudoir behavior, your husband is having a revelation. "Hey, maybe I've got something here," he thinks. The next thing you know, he's dragging you off for a shopping spree at Frederick's of Hollywood. Okay, maybe your old nighttime uniform of flannel boxers and a stained 5K Turkey Trot T-shirt wasn't necessarily in the sensual sleepwear category. Although Frederick's may not be your jammies of choice, don't let your husband's idea of romance frustrate you. Men are much more visual, so if you're okay with slipping into something more comfortable (clearly a man came up with this saying, as it is never "more comfortable"), we say give it a go.

We have a TTC who swears she'd rather wear a duck suit than anything with leather or lace. If you feel the same way about lingerie, be creative. Maybe you can spice things up with edible body paints or exotic oils. We know . . . you're immediately thinking, "How many times a week will I have to change the sheets if we get into body art?" Push that thought out of your mind. Once you release your inner artist, your husband may be more than willing to pick up the extra load of laundry.

The Sexsuit

To: Shelly <Shelly@conceptionchronicles.com>;
         Courtney <Courtney@conceptionchronicles.com>
From: Patty <Patty@conceptionchronicles.com>
Subject: **Victoria's Secret**

Victoria's secret is that she's not a mom or trying to be one!

I just got back from a shopping spree at Victoria's Secret. I was determined to get myself a "sexy" little number for this month's ovulation festivities. As I looked around the store, I had no interest in any of the merchandise displayed on the size 0 mannequins with perky breasts and pouty lips. I wanted the cute, fitted, cotton nightie with spaghetti straps and a built-in bra. In my pre-ovulation life this would have been fine, but now I feel like the stakes have been raised, and I keep giving in to the pressure.

That's when I realized this was not about me or what I wanted. Lingerie is just another part of the process, and, quite frankly, I find it as irritating as the stick or the thermometer. I ended up buying something that is undeniably in the "sexy" category—it's extremely uncomfortable and could double as a rock-climbing harness. I can't believe it's come to this. But if this is what it's going to take to get pregnant—strapping myself into something made of dental floss—I'll do it!

To: Patty <Patty@conceptionchronicles.com>;
          Shelly <Shelly@conceptionchronicles.com>
From: Courtney <Courtney@conceptionchronicles.com>
Subject: **The Sexsuit**

Slutty lingerie is one of the great mysteries of life. You would think having a baby should be inspired by good old-fashioned love. So how did one of the most beautiful moments in life become an amateur porn video staring yours truly, and why is your husband so excited about it? Does he really want the mother of his child to resemble the Whore of Babylon?

The good news is, when you finally do give birth, your memories of prancing around the bed in a French maid's uniform are quickly forgotten. So take advantage of your skimpy sexsuit while you can. It will soon be replaced with quick-release nursing bras and extra-large flannel jammies.

To: Patty <Patty@conceptionchronicles.com>;
          Courtney <Courtney@conceptionchronicles.com>
From: Shelly <Shelly@conceptionchronicles.com>
Subject: **RE: The Sexsuit**

Very impressive, Patty! Bruce is happy if I take off my sweat socks. I hope he and Scott don't start swapping stories.

We feel morally responsible to issue a warning about the sexsuit. While your husband is jumping for joy that the opportunity to "slut you up" has unexpectedly fallen in his lap, your short-term strategies may turn into long-term consequences. One of our TTCs who was trying for number two decided her new sex kitten look was just too much to handle with her busy schedule as the mother of a toddler. So she worked out a compromise with her husband. She would doll herself up one day a week for his viewing pleasure . . . and so, Slutty Saturday was born. What she failed to specify was she only planned to be a trampy pirate when she was ovulating. She created a monster. We're all convinced she'll be at the Shady Oaks retirement village, and her husband will pry himself off the oxygen machine just long enough for his favorite day of the week . . . *Slutty Saturday!*

The Secret Formula

Don't be surprised if you are completely exhausted after a few months of unlimited sex. The theoretical three-day fertile window has turned into a ten-day safety net sex marathon, and still you have nothing to show for it. What are you doing wrong? You've been diligently monitoring your ovulation; you're definitely having enough, and possibly on the brink of too much, sex; you've even affectionately named one of your fluffiest pillows "The Butt Booster" because you religiously prop yourself up after sex to help the sperm get where they need to go. So why aren't you pregnant?

Each passing month leaves you questioning your strategy. Did we have enough sex? Did we have too much sex? Did I have too much caffeine? Did that glass of wine at dinner lull his sperm into a slow-moving slumber? Talking to your inner circle of friends will only leave you feeling more confused. Their advice, which always comes along with a testimonial that they got pregnant in two months using their personal technique, varies from having sex every other day, to having sex twice a day, to our personal favorite, standing on your head for fifteen minutes after intercourse.

The problem is there is no magic formula for success. If there were, it would be packaged in a beautiful box and sold for $99.99 at every store across the country. Even when we pressed our doctors for advice about frequency of sex, they wouldn't commit. They said, "Every other day is sufficient." We tried that one month, and when we weren't successful, we decided we weren't striving for sufficient, we were striving for success. So we bypassed our trained medical professional's advice and went straight to our girlfriends. Next thing you knew, we were having a sunrise special and scouring garage sales for inversion boots.

The Monday-Morning Quarterback

The pressure to succeed may become too much to bear as the rules of the game change dramatically from month to month. Your constant pre-ovulation pep talks with your husband may lead to tension and flat-out rebellion on his part. He may just say enough is enough when you tell him he can still make his 7 A.M. breakfast meeting and keep to the ovulation schedule if you are both awake and ready to go by 4 A.M. the next morning.

Of course, if you skip even one day of sex and end up with a big fat negative, you will be unable to contain your annoyance at your husband for not "doing it" when you asked him. If only he would have listened to you, you'd be registering at Babies"R"Us instead of rummaging through your medicine cabinet in search of next month's supply of ovulation sticks.

Are You Going Too Far?

One day, your husband comes home and announces he will be attending a bachelor party in Las Vegas with a few of his buddies. Even though its four months away, you immediately think of your schedule and wonder if you'll be home alone ovulating as your husband is getting a lap dance at some seedy club. When you bring up your concerns—about the timing, not the lap dance—to your husband, he says you're crazy and insists everything cannot revolve around your ovulation. You have to continue to have a life.

Fine. You agree he should go to the bachelor party; after all, it is one of his dearest friends. But you also realize the tension around your pregame planning is really getting out of control. Your constant reminders of the status of your ovulation, coupled with e-mails to the office and voice mails on the cell phone, are getting to be too much. For the next few months before he heads off to viva Las Vegas, you will be a little more discreet about your ovulation.

Silence Is Deadly

After a few months of particularly high-stress sex on demand, some of our TTCs decided to try a new approach and keep their husbands completely in the dark about their bodily functions. Think this is taking it too far? If you find yourself sneaking ovulation sticks into the bathroom among an armful of fresh towels, odds are yes, you've gone too far.

However, keeping hubby out of the ovulation loop does have some distinct advantages:

1. No need to drag out the sexsuit. For all he knows it's just another day, so the flannel boxers are acceptable.
2. Seduction techniques can return to subtle eyebrow raising instead of a mass communications marketing blitz.
3. Husband does not complain of feeling "used" as you climb into bed.

You may be thinking there is no way you could pull off this sudden shift in strategy. Wouldn't your husband be suspicious if you flipped the calendar to a new month and didn't call a meeting to discuss the status of your cervical fluid? He certainly knows what your cycle day is today. Wouldn't he figure it out on his own? Surprisingly, regardless of how long you've been at this, if you don't take the lead like you always do, he will have no idea when you are ovulating and most likely won't ever bring it up. We promise he will not walk through the door one night and ask, "Honey, have you detected a surge in your luteinizing hormone?"

While the advantages of this approach are obvious, the potential pitfalls are a bit more subtle. Some of our TTCs claimed their husbands got so mad when they realized they had been suckered into service, they threatened to "skip it" for the next few months. You know it's serious if your husband willingly forfeits sex for the foreseeable future.

While your stealth strategy may reduce the initial tension around sex on demand, the end result is your husband is going to feel manipulated. So in good conscience, we feel compelled to issue a warning if you attempt this treacherous technique.

Pregnancy Is Pass/Fail

To:	Shelly <Shelly@conceptionchronicles.com>;
	Courtney <Courtney@conceptionchronicles.com>
From:	Patty <Patty@conceptionchronicles.com>
Subject:	**Results**

This month's efforts . . . very impressive, including a 1 a.m. sexathon with workaholic husband.

This month's results . . . negative!

At this point, you are no longer just exhausted, you're frustrated too. Something's got to give. You tell yourself you could have timed your ovulation better or had more sex or perhaps even tried a few more pieces of seductive clothing (you draw the line at tassels). But the reality is, you did everything you could, and you're still not pregnant.

Unfortunately, pregnancy is a pass/fail class. If only there were some way to indicate you were getting closer to achieving success. Wouldn't it be great if you received a report card at the end of each month detailing your performance . . . Effort: A+; Attitude: D; Human Sexuality: D; . . . final grade for Conception: F. The next month you would improve your attitude; study the Kama Sutra, which would ensure you an A+ in Human Sexuality; and pull your overall Conception grade up to a P (Pass/Pregnant).

Sorry, there are no report cards for those enrolled in Conception 101. You will never know if your constantly changing strategies, tracking devices and sexual frequency are getting you any closer to having a baby until one day you finally see a big pink line on the pregnancy stick.

What seems impossible is not. Remember when your brother gave you his Rubik's Cube with all the colors mixed, and you worked relentlessly for months to solve it to prove, without a doubt, you were the smartest one in the family? Were you really the smartest or the most tenacious? Pregnancy is the same way—it requires persistence. You just have to keep at it, twisting and turning and hoping that one month all the colors will align.

chapter four

The Fertile Friend

Tuesday	Notes

- Buy baby gifts for Sue, Kathi, Helen & Kim

- Restock liquor cabinet

Wednesday	Notes	Thursday	Notes

Just when you've convinced yourself getting pregnant is more a marathon than a sprint, the fertile friend appears. Every woman having trouble getting pregnant has a fertile friend. You know . . . the woman whose pregnancy is a "surprise." After spending so much time with your entire mind, body and soul dedicated to Operation Ovulation, you can't believe there are women out there who get pregnant without really trying. Sure, there was a time (not too long ago, in fact) when you thought it could just happen. But now you know what you know, and you are hard-pressed to believe women just wake up pregnant.

The stories you hear may vary from one woman to the next, but the theme is generally the same, and each tale leaves a bitter taste in your mouth. Not because your friend is pregnant and you are not, but because it seemed to happen so easily for her.

In case you haven't yet encountered a fertile friend, we've taken the liberty to characterize some of our favorites so they are instantly recognizable, and you can start practicing your Academy Award–winning performance of "Congratulations, I'm so thrilled for you."

We'd Like to Introduce You To . . .

The Odds Breaker (aka, the 1 Percent)

This is the friend you want with you when you're buying lottery tickets or picking long shots at the race track. However, when it comes to baby making, her luck at beating chemically controlled pregnancy probability is just too much to take. The Odds Breaker gets pregnant on the pill and swears she never missed a day. How come it worked for you all those years when you considered it a good week if you remembered to take the pill five out of seven days?

The Chosen

"We've been so blessed." In other words, God has chosen to bless this couple with children and not bless you and your husband. This is the thought that goes through your head each time you hear this woman tell someone she's pregnant. Does she believe God is looking down at your house from Heaven saying, "Sorry, try again next month."

The Professor

This woman has all the easy answers, whether you ask the questions or not. It's not a conversation with The Professor, but a lecture. Each time you talk with her, you feel like you're back in college when, no matter how much you studied, you never felt prepared for your accounting final exam. She insists if you would simply follow her lesson plan you'd be pregnant too.

The Bragger

"I'm so fertile, my husband just looks at me and I'm pregnant." We don't know a TTC out there who hasn't heard this one. The Bragger finally has her chance to let you know she is better than you—at something. You may be smarter, funnier and the superior golfer, but she gets the last laugh. She is definitely more fertile. Bitch.

The Lucky One

"The first time was a charm for us. We tried once, and it just happened." You've had perfectly orchestrated ovulation sex at least a thousand times and nothing. You thought the "first time" phenomenon only happened to fast, young girls who didn't listen to their mothers. Lucky or unlucky, life is just not fair.

The Networker

"It was really easy for ME to get pregnant, but I know someone who has a friend who has the same problem you seem to have . . . and they're pregnant. Just let me put you in touch with them." The Networker is invaluable when you're looking for a job or an apartment, but when it comes to baby making, she doesn't seem to understand your resistance in discussing your "trying" tribulations with her best friend's cousin's sister.

The Partier

"We were so drunk, I don't even remember having sex that night. I never thought sperm could survive so much tequila." This doesn't sound like moderation to you. Having a glass of wine is a major treat for you, and this lush gets pregnant doing body shots? You curse your strict beverage diet of water, freshly squeezed carrot juice and unsweetened decaffeinated tea.

The Virgin Mary

She says, "I really don't know how it happened." Is she serious? Sure, you may have been a little clueless about the ins and outs of all things ovulation when you first started trying, but you certainly knew *how* it happened.

No matter the fertile friend or the story she happens to be sharing, your initial gut reaction may not be exactly what you expect. Of course, you are genuinely happy for your friend, but you may also be embarrassed to admit you're feeling a little sad because it's not you. Who are you? You've never been one to be jealous of your friends or to use others as a benchmark for measuring your own life. You slap yourself on the wrist, push your pity party to the back of your mind and get back to the conversation at hand. After all, this is one of the most exciting moments in your friend's life, and you hope someday she can repay the favor by supporting you when you have good news to share.

Fertile Friend or Fertile Foe?

Like bubble gum, ice cream and beer, fertile friends come in an assortment of varieties and flavors. However, for simplicity's sake, there are really only two basic types you should be familiar with and understand: the friend and the foe. The fertile friends are your closest, best girlfriends. No matter how tactlessly they may break their good news or hand out their individual advice, they sincerely have your best interests at heart and are inspired from a genuine, good place.

On the contrary, the motivation behind the fertile foe can be downright questionable. These gleeful gals are typically just acquaintances, coworkers or family members whose relationship with you may be strained in one way or another. They seem to get some warped satisfaction out of the fact that they can get pregnant and you cannot. Be aware—and honest with yourself—about whether you are dealing with a fertile friend or a fertile foe. It will make all the difference in the world in coping with her behavior.

It's not always easy to tell the difference between a fertile friend and fertile foe, so we've developed a quick test to help you sharpen your detection skills:

1. Your friend knows you've been aggressively trying for more than a few months when she boastfully announces at a party she got pregnant the first month she and her husband tried. Answer: Foe

2. Your friend sends you her must-have fertility book, with a note expressing she hopes it brings the same success for you and your husband. Answer: Friend

3. Your friend calls to see if you can recommend a fertility specialist for her colleague since she obviously doesn't know one.
It doesn't seem to matter that you've never discussed with her
whether you're seeing a specialist. Answer: Foe

The ground rule for trying to figure out if you're dealing with a
fertile friend or fertile foe is to consider if you believe her intentions to be sincere, considerate and kind. If you think they are
authentic, then trust yourself—they likely are.

Fertile Friend Faux Pas

Remember, a fertile friend has no idea you're anything but happy
for her. Why would she think anything else? Because she is a bit
oblivious to your fertility-focused reality, she is destined for mis-
steps and mistakes. She's your friend and wants to pass on her
tricks for trying with you and frankly with any TTC who will
listen. Having experienced the joy of getting pregnant, it's only natural for a woman who has triumphed with a favorite fertility formula to be compelled to share it with ALL her friends who are
trying. The fertile friend simply thinks to herself, "Removing all
caffeine from my husband's diet worked for us, and if I share this
little tidbit, she'll get pregnant too." The TTC on the receiving end
of the advice thinks to herself, "You know I've been trying to get
pregnant forever; don't you think I've already tried that and everything else!?"

There are also fertile friend good deeds that can be wildly mis-
interpreted. One of our TTCs questioned the real impetus behind
her fertile friend's peculiar choice of gifts. After getting pregnant
herself, the fertile friend dropped off a giant care package filled
with unopened boxes of tampons, ovulation kits and pregnancy
tests. To our TTC, it was the most inconsiderate regifting she had

ever experienced. She felt her fertile friend was throwing in her face the fact that she no longer needed the goods but knew our TTC still did. It's likely the fertile friend genuinely believed she was doing something nice by passing them along and thought they would come in handy. Keep in mind, a fertile friend's penchant to help usually comes from a good place.

Please Stop Asking Me If I'm Pregnant

Another common fertile friend indiscretion is asking, "Are you pregnant?" in every conversation. What was previously a question born from thoughtful curiosity can now feel like a kick in the stomach each time you anticipate the query coming. Your pregnant pal probably wants you to share the joy she is feeling. To her, there would be no better way to do that than if you were pregnant too. Our advice here is to err on the side of caution and show a little restraint. While you may want to abruptly retort, "No, not yet!" before she even gets the words out of her mouth, we recommend turning your sweetness dial to ten and gently replying, "Trust me, you don't need to keep asking. I promise you'll be the first to know." Hopefully she will read between the lines and back off for a month or two.

Pity Party of One

If you are in the child-bearing age range, then chances are pretty good that a significant part of your social life now revolves around children, even if you don't have any of your own. Suddenly it seems like the only mail you get are coupon packs, catalogs and baby shower invitations. You're finding it difficult to admit, but you are definitely engrossed in a healthy dose of self-pity. Never before in your life do you recall feeling so sorry for yourself, but you do now, and it's not an emotion you're comfortable with. In the past, hearing about a friend's pregnancy always made you happy, but these days when you learn of another baby on the way, you are overcome with sadness and, at the same time, guilt for being so self-centered.

You remember when a baby shower invitation arrived in the mail, and it gave you a warm, happy feeling; you couldn't wait to check out the latest in bassinettes, bouncy seats and baby wear. Lately, when a little pink or blue envelope arrives, you seek advice on how to survive the shower without gorging yourself on the artichoke dip or drowning your sorrows in the mimosas instead of searching the mom-to-be's registry at PBKids.com. You imagine watching the mom-to-be open gift after gift of baby books and baby blankets, and it makes you wonder if you can make it through without losing your mind. If you fantasize about the moment when some innocent guest inevitably asks, "Are you trying?" and secretly to yourself you reply, "Me? No. I hate children," then it may be time to send your regrets and stay home.

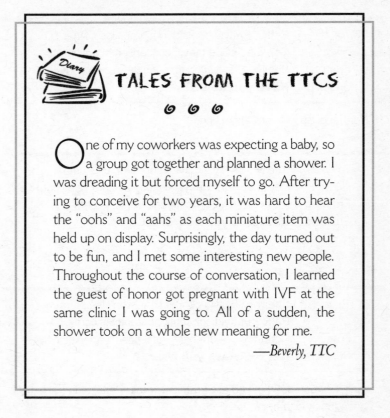

TALES FROM THE TTCS

One of my coworkers was expecting a baby, so a group got together and planned a shower. I was dreading it but forced myself to go. After trying to conceive for two years, it was hard to hear the "oohs" and "aahs" as each miniature item was held up on display. Surprisingly, the day turned out to be fun, and I met some interesting new people. Throughout the course of conversation, I learned the guest of honor got pregnant with IVF at the same clinic I was going to. All of a sudden, the shower took on a whole new meaning for me.

—*Beverly, TTC*

You have to take each invitation and each day as they come. Some days you will be more than happy to join in on the shower games, while others, the thought of unscrambling twenty baby names may be enough to send you over the edge. On these days, a nice gift and a thoughtful note will go a long way to save both your sanity and your relationships.

To: Patty <Patty@conceptionchronicles.com>;
           Courtney <Courtney@conceptionchronicles.com>
From: Shelly <Shelly@conceptionchronicles.com>
Subject: **Have you heard?**

Tom and his wife are expecting.

To: Shelly <Shelly@conceptionchronicles.com>;
           Courtney <Courtney@conceptionchronicles.com>
From: Patty <Patty@conceptionchronicles.com>
Subject: **RE: Have you heard?**

No . . . But that's such great news!

To: Shelly <Shelly@conceptionchronicles.com>;
           Patty <Patty@conceptionchronicles.com>
From: Courtney <Courtney@conceptionchronicles.com>
Subject: **RE: RE: Have you heard?**

Isn't it awesome? I talked to Sarah last week. Patty, didn't you just have lunch with her?

To: Patty <Patty@conceptionchronicles.com>;
           Courtney <Courtney@conceptionchronicles.com>
From: Shelly <Shelly@conceptionchronicles.com>
Subject: **RE: RE: RE: Have you heard?**

Patty, I'm sure she didn't mention it to you because she thought it might upset you.

To:	Shelly <Shelly@conceptionchronicles.com>; Courtney <Courtney@conceptionchronicles.com>
From:	Patty <Patty@conceptionchronicles.com>
Subject:	**RE: RE: RE: RE: Have you heard?**

Are you kidding me? I couldn't be happier for them.

So what? Now, because I'm not pregnant, I'm only going to be receiving bad news? I guess my phone will only ring when there's a death, divorce or terminal illness.

Can a Fertile Friend Still Be a Friend?

It's likely your fertile friends are wondering how to handle this new awkwardness that stands between you and your friendship. Remember, they really do have your best interests at heart, so be sure you thank them for their ongoing support, and let them know how much it means to you. It's also important to reiterate how truly happy you are for them and their pregnancies. It will mean the world to your fertile friend if you can share the joy at this special time of her life. The best thing you can do is have a heart-to-heart talk with her and honestly discuss the situation—both yours and hers. Come to an agreement that you are both comfortable with how you want to talk about her pregnancy and about your efforts at trying to conceive. Suggest you'd like to take the lead when it comes to your efforts in the bedroom and emphasize that you know she'll be thinking about you even if she isn't asking, "Are you pregnant?" every time you chat.

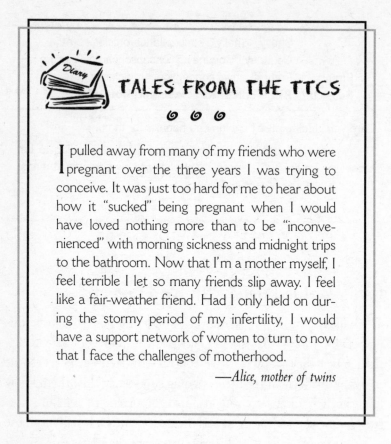

TALES FROM THE TTCS

I pulled away from many of my friends who were pregnant over the three years I was trying to conceive. It was just too hard for me to hear about how it "sucked" being pregnant when I would have loved nothing more than to be "inconvenienced" with morning sickness and midnight trips to the bathroom. Now that I'm a mother myself, I feel terrible I let so many friends slip away. I feel like a fair-weather friend. Had I only held on during the stormy period of my infertility, I would have a support network of women to turn to now that I face the challenges of motherhood.

—*Alice, mother of twins*

The Fertile Foe

Unfortunately, fertile foes are more adversaries than advocates in your struggle to get pregnant. It's a sad yet simple fact that women are not always nice to other women. And among some, there lies an undercurrent of fundamental competitiveness, even when it's something as sacred as trying to have a baby. Again, this is more likely to surface or ensue among acquaintances or in strained relationships and not with your true friends. Yet we've had TTCs tell us their most honest reaction to a fertile foe's pregnancy still left them completely horrified; they were embarrassed to admit it, but they felt like the fertile foes were turning getting pregnant into a competition.

The underlying issue may be that today's women are driven, successful and maniacally focused on getting the results they want, when they want them. When we set our minds to accomplish something, we get it done. Whether it's graduating from college with honors (or just trying to finish), finding the ideal mate (or a nice guy with all of his hair), landing a dream job (or one that pays the bills), we feel we are in complete control of our lives. You may start to realize getting pregnant is the one challenge where you have little influence over the outcome.

Managing your expectations may become a long-term problem if you don't get pregnant right away, especially if you are viewing each foe's pregnancy as a point lost for you. So put away the scorecard, and just keep your focus where it belongs . . . on yourself.

Surviving Fertile Foes

While it would be awfully nice to avoid a fertile foe at all costs during her pregnancy and while you are trying, there are many circumstances that will not allow it. Distancing yourself is not always an option, especially if the fertile foe is a family member or coworker. Unfortunately, like dandelions and crab grass, annoying fertile foes also grow close to home. And when a cousin, coworker or boss is starring in the role, you can expect hurt feelings and anger to run deep. Our advice is to revert back to your Girl Scout days and remember their motto—Be Prepared. Wait a minute, that was the Boy Scout motto, but it works here too. When dealing with fertile foes, your best defense is a good offense. Try to be prepared for anything, but even when they continue to shock you with their insensitive remarks, take the high road.

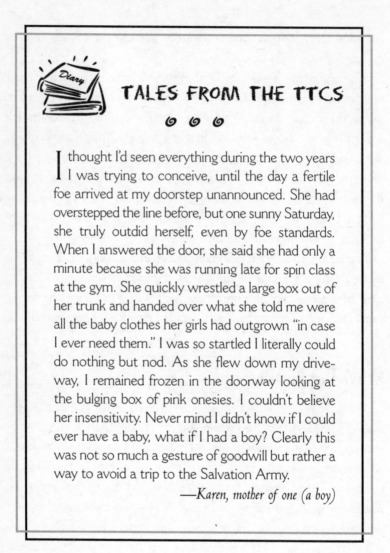

TALES FROM THE TTCS

I thought I'd seen everything during the two years I was trying to conceive, until the day a fertile foe arrived at my doorstep unannounced. She had overstepped the line before, but one sunny Saturday, she truly outdid herself, even by foe standards. When I answered the door, she said she had only a minute because she was running late for spin class at the gym. She quickly wrestled a large box out of her trunk and handed over what she told me were all the baby clothes her girls had outgrown "in case I ever need them." I was so startled I literally could do nothing but nod. As she flew down my driveway, I remained frozen in the doorway looking at the bulging box of pink onesies. I couldn't believe her insensitivity. Never mind I didn't know if I could ever have a baby, what if I had a boy? Clearly this was not so much a gesture of goodwill but rather a way to avoid a trip to the Salvation Army.

—Karen, mother of one (a boy)

TALES FROM THE TTCS

🌀 🌀 🌀

Fertile foes are not reserved for those trying for their first baby. I have a four-year-old daughter and have been trying to give her a sibling for longer than I care to remember. One day, I was at a play date with a woman who had three children and another on the way. This foe, who knew I'd love nothing more than a Brady Bunch–sized family said, "We'd love to have Amy spend the night, but I just don't think she'd do well at our house." When I asked her what she meant, she replied, "Well, we just have so many kids running around; our family may be too hectic for her." I found myself trying to justify that my daughter was used to plenty of commotion since she is always playing with her cousins and other kids. It's not as if I keep her locked in the basement. But what I really wanted to say was, there may be only three of us, but we're a family too.

—*Diane, mother of one*

Spin the Wheel of Emotion

How you will react to a fertile friend or fertile foe will most likely depend on where you are in the process of trying to conceive. If it's still early, you are likely to find it very easy to be happy for a fertile friend who gets pregnant before you do, and a fertile foe's rude remarks or insensitive innuendo will be lost on you. However, as time marches on, you may become more anxious about your own ability to conceive. An irritating sensation can replace your carefree confidence that things will work out. And while it's okay to be worried and feel a little sorry for yourself, don't lose hope or sight of the options that may lie ahead. The road to motherhood may be prolonged, and too much self-pity and self-doubt will make the trip impossible to tolerate. As hard as it may be, you have to find the strength to be optimistic and remain focused on your end goal—having a child.

Even Rainy Days Have a Purpose

Every living creature has a significant purpose in continuing the circle of life, and the same holds true for each friend in your fertility sphere. It may not be clear to you at first, but a fertile friend or foe can play a valuable role in your continuing quest for motherhood. She may be the catalyst that forces you to take an honest look at where you are in the process of trying to conceive and gives you the nudge you need to seek the help of a doctor. Two years from now, she may turn out to be the one who gives you advice on 2 A.M. feedings and tips for getting your baby to sleep through the night.

chapter five

Calling in the Pros

Friday   Notes

- *Remind hubby of fertility specialist appt.*

Saturday   Notes   **Sunday**   Notes

- *Remind hubby of fertility specialist appt.*

- *Fertility specialist appt. 3 P.M.*

Your fertile friends are producing offspring faster than your sixth-grade pet hamsters. You've never been one to believe in symbolism or signs, but maybe all of these pregnant pals are appearing out of the woodwork for a reason. The pesky feeling you've had in the back of your mind has moved center stage, and you are fairly certain the amount of time you've spent trying to get pregnant has surpassed normal. You wanted to get pregnant on your own, and until now you truly believed you could . . . and would. Now you begin to question yourself and your body. Patience is a virtue, but in your case it may be a vice as it's preventing you from dealing with the truth.

This month is different. You're without answers after you get your period . . . again. You look at yourself in the mirror and see its time to face reality—you need "professional help."

You Know It's Time to See a Specialist When . . .

You can't remember the last time you took a birth control pill or a moment when you didn't know the exact day of your cycle. You keep repeating the "unwritten rule" in your head. If you're under thirty-five and have been trying to conceive for more than a year or over thirty-five and have been trying for six months, it's time to seek the help of a doctor. You begin recalling bits and pieces of a conversation with a friend who told you she was seeing a fertility specialist. While you listened intently to her story at the time, you never banked the details of her experience, not because you weren't interested, but because you never believed it would apply to you.

Damn it. You can perfectly recite from memory her grandma's secret recipe for fried chicken and dumplings, but for the life of you, you simply can't recall the name of the fertility doctor she saw.

Hearing the Words, "You Need a Specialist"

Like any problem, the first step to resolving it is admitting you actually have one. Regardless of your age, how long you've been trying or if this is your first or fourth child, hearing you need to see a specialist will, no doubt, leave you breathless.

It's incredibly difficult to admit you may have fertility issues, but try to keep things in perspective. You are trying to have a baby and simply need the advice and assistance of a doctor. While it's an unexpected hurdle, acknowledging you need to see a specialist can be a real relief. You know the sooner you figure out what you can do to increase your chances of pregnancy, the closer you'll be to motherhood. However, anxiety creeps in, as you cannot imagine what could possibly be wrong.

To: Courtney <Courtney@conceptionchronicles.com>;
           Shelly <Shelly@conceptionchronicles.com>
From: Patty <Patty@conceptionchronicles.com>
Subject: **Yikes!**

I went in for my annual OB-GYN appointment this morning and mentioned I've been trying to get pregnant with no luck. When my doctor asked me how long we've been trying, I told her it's been almost a year. Then she asked me how old I was. I jokingly answered, "I'm 35 and 11/12," but I didn't get the chuckle I expected. Instead, she put on her most serious medical face and said I needed to find a specialist.

Do you really think it's necessary?

To:	Patty <Patty@conceptionchronicles.com>
From:	Shelly <Shelly@conceptionchronicles.com>
Cc:	Courtney <Courtney@conceptionchronicles.com>
Subject:	**RE: Yikes!**

Do they make Hallmark cards for an 11/12 birthday? Might not be a bad idea; at the very least start looking for a referral.

To:	Patty <Patty@conceptionchronicles.com>
From:	Courtney <Courtney@conceptionchronicles.com>
Cc:	Shelly <Shelly@conceptionchronicles.com>
Subject:	**RE: RE: Yikes!**

I agree with Shelly—it can't hurt to see a specialist. I doubt there's anything wrong, but at least you'll cover all your bases.

There's No Problem Here . . . Just Move Along, Folks

Just because you've accepted it's time to seek fertility help, don't expect a similar outward reaction from your husband. He may not embrace the same attitude, at least not in the beginning. Women are usually the first ones to admit there is a problem because we live it day in and day out. We ride the roller coaster every month, only to have it crescendo with the relentless reminder of a five-day menstrual cycle. And while they may not be sitting shotgun, our husbands' moods are reflective of our constantly changing highs and lows.

When it comes to their own health, most men are bigger babies than the newborns we hope to one day deliver. Despite your husband's typical hypochondriac behavior (he gets a common cold and thinks he needs the urgent care wing of the nearest hospital), be prepared for his inability to comprehend the possibility of malfunctioning reproductive equipment. And that's if he thinks you have the problem. Heaven forbid his manhood is called into question.

Your husband may still be in the "we don't have a problem, we just need to have more sex" frame of mind. Operation Ovulation has turned your three fertile days into twelve, and you can't imagine when you could possibly squeeze in extra sex. You wish it were that simple.

Like the passenger in a sidecar, he's clearly along for the ride just to appease you—first, because he probably has no idea what the words reproductive endocrinologist mean, and second, because he will be extremely concerned about his role in the process. If you find your husband floundering in the waters of denial and panic, toss him a lifeline and pull him back to the shores of reality. You're going to need him.

Is There a Doctor in the House?

You may be the kind of woman who wades slowly into chilly waters—dipping in one foot at a time, gently easing your body, limb by limb, into the depths before completely submerging yourself. Although your goal is to minimize the shock, you are most likely prolonging the agony. Or maybe you're a bold soul who dives headfirst into the deep end without so much as testing the temperature with your big toe. If you get a rush from taking things head on, then finding a good specialist may be a relatively easy process for you. But if you're more patient and contemplative in your approach, the process of finding Dr. Right may take you a bit longer.

No matter your speed or style, selecting the right specialist can be a completely overwhelming process. Tons of questions are running through your head as you struggle to understand where you should even begin. What *is* a reproductive endocrinologist? How do I find one? Are the Yellow Pages an option? We recommend building a qualified pool of doctors from a variety of reliable sources.

A good place to start is to ask your own OB-GYN for a referral. It's likely that your doctor has a specialist he or she typically recommends to patients. You might also consider reaching out to those friends in your inner circle who have been through fertility treatment. There are obvious success stories among them based on the fleet of Maclaren Rally Twin Strollers you've seen them pushing around.

The World Wide Web is the next logical place when searching for referrals. The American Society for Reproductive Medicine (ASRM) Web site can offer information about finding a certified doctor in your area as well as help answer some of the questions you may have.

When picking a specialist, your first inclination may be to find one who is convenient. Patty found her *first* specialist because she limited her search to doctors in the same zip code. Big mistake. Despite the convenient location, the doctor and Patty were not the right fit at all. Precious months were wasted as she and her doctor never connected, and Patty was ultimately forced to find another specialist.

Pray Short-term, Plan Long-term

After collecting the names of specialists from your OB-GYN, your friends and the Internet, a crucial step in finding the right doctor is to check each doctor's credentials. The Centers for Disease Control's (CDC) Web site is an incredible place to find exactly what you'll need and want to know about each doctor's results with assisted reproduction—primarily IVF (in vitro fertilization)—patients. And while you may be nowhere near considering IVF, it's best to plan long-term as if IVF may become an option for you one day. The level of success rates can be a helpful gauge and indicator to consider when comparing doctors and clinics.

So while you're finishing your morning coffee and checking your inbox, spend the extra time you need to fully research the fertility specialists you are considering.

Mid-forties Specialist with Great Results Seeks Woman Trying to Conceive

After you've completed your research and narrowed down your list to the doctors with good success rates, the next critical step is to meet with each doctor in person. If you've ever looked for love via the Internet or answered a personal ad, you know that most people look better on paper than in person. So whether the referral comes from a friend, the Web or your OB-GYN, you need to feel completely comfortable with your doctor, and the best way to establish a good match is to meet with several before selecting one. Like a great pair of heels, a fertility specialist needs to fit just right.

And if you have your mind set on a female specialist, you should know that most reproductive endocrinologists tend to be men. So if you've always frequented female OB-GYNs, then you need to open your mind to the possibility that a male doctor could be your conduit to motherhood.

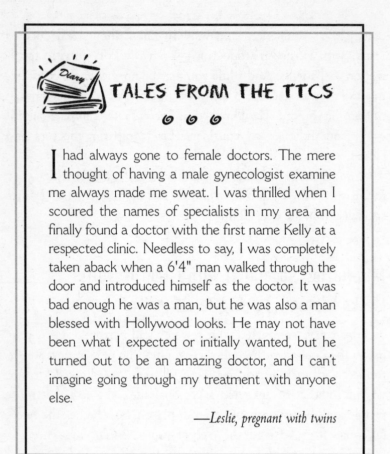

TALES FROM THE TTCS

I had always gone to female doctors. The mere thought of having a male gynecologist examine me always made me sweat. I was thrilled when I scoured the names of specialists in my area and finally found a doctor with the first name Kelly at a respected clinic. Needless to say, I was completely taken aback when a 6'4" man walked through the door and introduced himself as the doctor. It was bad enough he was a man, but he was also a man blessed with Hollywood looks. He may not have been what I expected or initially wanted, but he turned out to be an amazing doctor, and I can't imagine going through my treatment with anyone else.

—Leslie, pregnant with twins

Please Don't Answer

You've decided on your specialist and found the courage to make the call and schedule your first appointment. At precisely twelve noon, you dial the phone but silently pray no one answers. They should be closed for lunch, right? You rationalize you should get credit just for making the call. When someone promptly answers, you almost hang up. Evidently, Nurse Ratched has decided to eat her tuna salad at her desk today. A rush of panic washes over you as the nurse asks if you're calling about INFERTILITY issues. A dialogue ensues:

Nurse: Doctor's office, please hold. [ten minutes pass]
You: Yes, I'm calling about my FERTILITY issues.
Nurse: Have you sought help for INFERTILITY in the past?
You: No, this is the first time I'm contacting a FERTLITY specialist.
Nurse: Well then, we'll need to send you our INFERTILITY information packet. What's your address?
You: You can send the FERTILITY packet to 521 Candlewood Lane.
Nurse: We'll need the INFERTILITY worksheet completed and returned before your first appointment.

Uncle.

You begin to robotically answer her questions, but at the same time you feel frustrated and angry. Why is this happening to you? You start playing mind games with yourself. If I give myself just a little more time, I'll be pregnant. Maybe I rushed too quickly to see a specialist, and this call is a sign it wasn't meant to be. Maybe my husband is right, and I'm overreacting. You tell yourself if the nurse says "infertility" one more time, it's game over and you are hanging up. You hope she gives you the out.

No such luck. She schedules an appointment weeks from now and tells you she'll mail the welcome packet to you today. What exactly are you being welcomed to—the infertility club? This is one society you never wanted to join.

For those of you who enjoy instant gratification, be prepared— you will not get it anywhere in the fertility treatment process. It can be eight to twelve weeks from the time you schedule your appointment until the time you meet with your doctor face-to-face. After all the buildup to make the appointment, you are relieved to know it's not for a few months. At least the date is on your calendar.

Maybe you'll be pregnant by then anyway.

You wax and wane between feeling excited about your appointment and apprehensive when you think about what might be wrong with you. The good news is there are many treatment options available to couples once the correct diagnosis is provided.

If You're Going to Be Naked, You're Going to Need Coverage

Before you explore your fertility options, you should fully investigate your insurance coverage and review the out-of-pocket costs associated with the various treatments. Going through fertility treatment will be far less stressful if you know in advance the details of your coverage. And if you find your insurance company does not cover certain tests or treatments, you can prepare financially. Make note of open enrollment dates and deadlines that may give you the ability to change or improve your benefits.

Some questions to think about: Which procedures and drug therapies are covered? Are there age restrictions? Are there financial caps? What benefits are included, and what are excluded? We know navigating the minutiae of insurance policies can be overwhelming, but it's a necessary evil when the possibility of fertility treatment lies ahead. Hopefully, you will never need to rely on your insurance company for aggressive fertility benefits, but if you do, gathering as much information now may help you make difficult decisions later.

Preappointment "Welcome" Packet

You try to block out your looming appointment, that is, until the welcome packet arrives. The support you're expecting from your husband shines through as he tosses the packet on the kitchen table and says, "This is definitely yours." So much for sharing in the process. You rip open the oversized envelope, and out drops a brochure for the clinic. A woman caressing her newborn is staring right at you; the caption gently promises: "Where Dreams Come True." As you dump the contents of the packet onto the table (being sure to cover up the mother and baby), you wonder how you will ever get through the pages of information by the time your appointment arrives. You were expecting a fairly routine set of questions regarding your menstrual cycle and how long you've been trying to conceive. You weren't completely prepared for the brochure that welcomes you into the arms of fertility treatment.

You feel like you are taking entrance exams all over again, but the stakes are much higher at "Fertility U." You may feel besieged and beleaguered as you begin to answer the surplus of questions about your medical and sexual history. This is no time to exaggerate or hold back on any details. You are uncomfortable just thinking about answering the questions in the privacy of your own home and dread the thought of discussing them with a stranger. You're no prude, and you've been known to have candid sexual conversations with your girlfriends, especially after a couple of glasses of wine. Now it's time to have the same conversation with a man in a white coat, and you want to run for cover.

Forget the Cosmo Quiz. These questions are not about finding your sexual soul mate or getting to your g-spot. It's facts and figures here, although there may be one or two questions that throw you for a curve.

- Do you have sex with multiple partners? *Hell no, I have a hard enough time having sex with my husband before, during and after ovulation. When would I fit in a lover?*
- Does your husband masturbate? *I don't know when he'd find the time, but good for him if he still has energy to burn.*
- Have you experienced a sudden weight loss or gain in the last

six months? Yes, but I assume it's my addiction to Rocky Road and Chunky Monkey and has nothing to do with my hormones running amok.

To Go or Not to Go: Your Husband's Role

Your husband may be amazed that you have actually made the appointment, as he still thinks you are overreacting. Remind him you are seeking the help of a specialist to move you closer to having a child. When considering whether your husband should attend the first appointment, most of our TTCs agreed that two sets of ears are better than one. You may have led the charge alone up to this point, but now is not the time to be brave. Save that for later. Take your husband with you, if only to have a hand to hold under the table. The best way to prepare your husband for his first foray into the world of fertility treatment is to give him a good, old-fashioned pep talk, and have him practice saying "masturbation," "vagina" and "ejaculation" with a straight face.

Every Journey Begins with One Small Step; You're Gonna Need the Right Shoes

So the big day has arrived. You have developed a love-hate relationship with this moment since making the appointment. As you prepare to step into uncharted fertility treatment waters, you are suddenly consumed with such inane details as what you should wear. First impressions count, and like any important appointment, you want to convey a certain image. For some strange reason, you are compelled to unmistakably project the aura of a loving, nurturing, maternal being. We can't tell you exactly what to wear, but we can definitely tell you what to avoid. Dark business suit screams, "I have been far too busy with my career to think about having children." Hot pink Juicy Couture sweatsuit with "Juicy" boldly written across the ass shouts, "I have worked out and dieted myself down to an anovulatory state." Oversized, faded T-shirt with gym shorts and sneakers bellows, "I'm unconscious and irresponsible and likely to leave a child unattended in a vehicle." It may not be the most important thing, but deciding what to wear in advance will save you time and stress as you get ready for your appointment.

Once inside the waiting room, you try to relax by reading outdated issues of *Time* magazine. You continually steal a glance at the couples checking in with the receptionist. You know you shouldn't, but you can't help but compare yourself with and evaluate your "competition." As you eye every woman walking into the clinic, each is clutching her "Where Dreams Come True" packet. Your inner dialogue begins, "More fertile. . . . Definitely more fertile. . . . Much less fertile. Younger. . . . Really young. . . . Much older." And so on. As much as you want to, try not to draw comparisons between any of the patients. You won't see one common thread among any of these women—infertility does not discriminate. Just when you've given up, the happy couple arrives. They are giggling, lost in their own world. Yes, they are giddy, and yes, they are pregnant! There is hope.

Your name is finally called, and you are led into the doctor's office. You and your husband exchange uncomfortable glances, and for a moment it seems you are a team and totally committed to one another and your dream of having a child. Then his cell phone rings, and as he starts to answer it, you wrestle it from his hands and without hesitation shut it off. You can't believe he was actually going to take the call. Moron. The doctor finally arrives; he is not at all what you expected. You were hoping for a gentle, bespectacled man with a smile that would make your worries disappear. Instead, the man standing in front of you looks like a Phi Delta Theta you dated back in college, minus the jumbo mug of beer. Take a deep breath and remember, he is here to help.

At this point, you'll probably walk your doctor through your entire medical history. It actually feels good to talk about your situation, and some of your frustrations feel like they are being lifted just by saying the words, "We are struggling." When you finish, your doctor nods and says, "Yes, you need to be here." Until that very moment, you were convinced he would tell you not to worry and send you on your way for another six months of trying. Not the case. Instead, he begins describing the litany of tests that begins the diagnostic process. Once the tests have been conducted and a diagnosis is made, he will recommend a treatment option. As he begins explaining the details around each treatment option, you fade in and out. You are suddenly transported to your favorite Italian restaurant, Mario's. It's Tuesday, so the special is penne with pancetta. You fixate on the word "pancetta." Is that Italian bacon or ham? Do I eat pancetta, or is it prosciutto that I like? It's not until the doctor asks if you have any questions that you snap back to reality. You haven't heard a single word since he said, "You need to be here."

If you're like us, our doctors utter one word or phrase that captures our attention and we end up focused on it at the expense of missing everything else. Having your husband along will ensure he is hearing the doctor's both optimistic and realistic observations as well as following along when you find yourself lost at Mario's for a moment or two.

Three Strikes and You're Out

The doctor lays out the basic treatments and explains, in most cases, the female infertility treatment process is a three-step program. You get three attempts at each step before "flunking out" and moving on to the next stage.

- Step One: Clomid
- Step Two: Injections/IUI (Intrauterine Insemination)
- Step Three: IVF

You've Only Just Begun

As you exit the clinic, your mind is racing with what your life is going to be like for the next few months. Meanwhile, your husband seems relatively unfazed as he scrolls down the missed calls list on his cell phone. By the time you reach the car, tears have welled in your eyes. He knows something is wrong, but in his attempts to soothe and comfort you, he can't quite figure out why you are so upset. As you try to explain, you can't. It's everything about the process that has you overwhelmed, embarrassed and scared. You fear your chances of having a baby are diminishing.

You shouldn't feel this way, as you are now on your way to figuring out what's wrong and doing something about it. And while you never thought fertility treatment would play a role in your efforts to conceive, you are inching closer to your dreams of having a child by taking this enormous first step.

chapter six

The Angry Ovulator

Monday

Notes

- Out of town!
- Ovulating

Tuesday

Notes

- Hubby traveling!!

Wednesday

Notes

- Sign up for
  mind/body
  yoga class

O Solo Mio—Why Do I Feel So Alone?

You're beginning to feel like the entire burden of conceiving a child is on you and you alone. When you made the decision to start a family, you understood the nine months you would actually be pregnant the responsibility of nurturing your child would primarily fall on you—your husband couldn't really help much in this area. However, you never thought the act of *trying to get pregnant* could make you feel so isolated. This was the part you would do together. But now that you're seeing a fertility specialist, it's becoming more and more obvious you may be on your own for much of the ride to motherhood.

Your mind is whirling with the times, dates and lab locations for the onslaught of tests you must endure. Trying to wedge these unplanned appointments into a schedule that's already packed with commuting, careers and commitments can seem almost impossible, but you know you'll figure out a way to juggle it all—you always do. Of course, there's really no need for your husband to accompany you to these appointments, and taking time off work is just as hard for him. So rather than disrupting two schedules, you'll go it alone. You can feel the resentment starting to build, but you push it out of your mind and tell yourself you're being ridiculous. What more could the poor guy do? After all, you're the one with the vagina.

If you could just get pregnant this month, you could forget the whole conception process and go back to your normal life. Your new doctor is nice enough, but you fantasize daily about calling him to let him know, as it turns out, you won't be coming back next month as planned. His services are no longer required—you've gotten pregnant the good old-fashioned way.

Why Can't I Ovulate on the Weekend?

The pressure continues to build as you move closer and closer to your ovulation date. You were almost getting used to the craziness of Operation Ovulation, but this month has much more serious consequences. If things don't work out, it won't be just you and your husband sharing your disappointment over a plate of fajitas at your favorite Mexican restaurant. No, a team of medical experts will critique this month's efforts. There's no way you're walking into their office and admitting you actually didn't have sex the day before you ovulated. First of all, you'll feel like a complete idiot, and second, why consult a team of experts if you aren't doing the basics at home? You vow this cycle will be perfect, and you will have as much sex as possible to cover an unplanned early or late ovulation.

Of course, this is always easier said than done. It is a known fact, regardless of your cycle, you will ovulate on every major holiday and every day that requires an out-of-town trip for you or your husband. In case there was ever a question, this proves without a shadow of a doubt the fertility gods have been blessed with a good sense of humor. So once again, you will be spinning out of control, rescheduling flights and trying to figure out how you will possibly have sex while at Aunt Sheila's Thanksgiving extravaganza.

In the old days, you would settle for coming home for the holidays a day late and leaving a day early. You'd do your best to squeeze in a quickie if the opportunity presented itself, but you didn't make yourself crazy. Those days are over. Now you're obsessed . . . and you should be. You can no longer afford to put others first. You and your ovulation are the number one priority, and nothing can stand in your way or hinder your efforts.

To:	Patty <Patty@conceptionchronicles.com>;
	Courtney <Courtney@conceptionchronicles.com>
From:	Shelly <Shelly@conceptionchronicles.com>
Subject:	**Uh "O" Overnight Guests**

Our attempts for number two were dampened a bit last night when Bruce announced an unexpected overnight guest. Any other time of the month I would have fluffed the pillows and baked a casserole, but I couldn't help feeling irritated. My ovulation is quickly approaching, and we should be having sex for the next two weeks. Sounds crazy, but you know the drill. Our walls are simply too thin, not to mention Maré would be sleeping a foot away from our bed so we could make room for our visitor. This wouldn't bother Bruce at all, but I, on the other hand, don't want our daughter humping her stuffed animals. Why am I the only one who seems to care?

To:	Shelly <Shelly@conceptionchronicles.com>
From:	Courtney <Courtney@conceptionchronicles.com>
Cc:	Patty <Patty@conceptionchronicles.com>
Subject:	**Avoiding Years of Therapy**

Be careful. Maré will be dumped out of day care faster than you can say "child services" if she starts demonstrating her new-found skills at school!

Like bees to a begonia, so too are overnight guests drawn to an ovulatory house. Friends you have not seen in years will suddenly appear for long weekends. And it's not just friends. Long-lost relatives will suddenly plan the trip "back East" they've been talking about for years and will, of course, stay with you as they tour the local sites. Think you can't say no? Think again. Of course, you must intercept the self-inviters before they reach your husband or you're doomed. Ovulation is the furthest thing from his mind, so without another thought he will say, "Sounds great," and the next thing you know your calendar is booked solid for the next two months.

If you're lucky enough to have a large house with a separate wing for drop-in guests, by all means open your arms to the masses. But if space is at a premium, you may want to reconsider. When you're not ovulating, everything seems possible with a pull-out couch. But be realistic. Do you really want Uncle Fred in the next room when you dust off the sexsuit and get busy?

Wake Me When It's Over

Even if you're lucky enough to keep your house guest-free during your ovulation, you will never be fortunate enough to ovulate on the weekend—that is, until you are undergoing serious medical treatment that requires an office visit during ovulation, and the offices are not open on Saturday or Sunday. Only then will your body instantly shift to ovulating only on weekends . . . but more about that later.

Wouldn't it be great to wake up on a sunny Saturday afternoon, enjoy a leisurely cup of decaf with the hubby and cruise the headline news before gearing up for a session of sex on demand? It will never happen. You will always ovulate in the middle of the craziest week you can imagine, and then you will be forced to squeeze in sex between dropping off the dry cleaning, paying past-due bills online and heading to the office for an early morning meeting. It's easy to see how your quest for a baby has started to turn into a real hassle. Sex is just another thing that must get done in an already overbooked day. You may be only twenty-five, thirty or forty, but ovulation makes you feel ready to apply for Social Security. You're just so tired of it all.

There's a New Emotion in Town

By the time you finally hit your fertile window, you are consumed with unfiltered, unabridged anger, and guess who the lucky recipient is to bear the wrath of your rage? That's right, it's the man you swore to love in good times and bad.

Why are you so angry? You're angry because life as you knew it is on hold. You'll get back to volunteering . . . once you get pregnant. You'll refocus at work . . . next month. You'll skip the second glass of wine at dinner . . . just in case. You'll start working out again . . . after the baby comes. All these things make you angry, but most of all, you're angry because you're still not pregnant. Literally, every aspect of your life is affected by your attempts to have a baby while your husband's life goes on as normal. He's working, hitting the gym, enjoying that extra beer and meeting friends for poker. Aside from having a lot more sex, things are basically status quo for him.

Your husband isn't the only one adding to your angst. If one more fertile friend tells you to "just relax and you'll be pregnant in no time," you're going to lose it. You've heard the story over and over, about so-and-so's cousin who was told she could never conceive a child, so she adopted and guess what? Of course, we all know what happened next . . . she got pregnant . . . on her own . . . without even seeing a doctor. Hurray for her! You paste an intrigued look on your face while using every ounce of energy you have left to suppress your primal urge to tackle this woman to the ground and beat the smugness out of her. If you weren't wearing your nice pants, you'd do it.

You can't wait for this torture to be over. Prayers to God no longer start with hopes for world peace. You've limited your request to one: "Please, please, please, God, let me get pregnant this month."

It's Not Just Like Riding a Bike

A mom who's trying to get pregnant again may be surprised by the mixed bag of emotions she feels as the process drags on. It may have been fairly easy for you to conceive the first time, so you initially wonder what's different? What's changed? Yes, you're a little older, but you'd always heard getting pregnant the second time was a lot easier, especially if you had a healthy pregnancy and an easy childbirth experience. You're doing everything you did the last time—and more—yet the plus sign remains elusive with each pregnancy test you take.

Like most mothers, you feel incredibly blessed to have a healthy child to call your own. However, as the unsuccessful months unfold, it may become hard on the ears and heart to hear a family member or close friend "comfort" you with such ridiculous reassurances as: "You should feel lucky to have one child. There are so many women who can't even have that." Since when did wanting more than one child become a selfish proposition? Is it so terrible to want a little brother or sister to play in the sandbox with Junior?

On top of the emotional highs and lows you're experiencing this time around, you may also be harboring feelings of guilt about how much energy and time you're putting toward trying to conceive and at what cost to your kids who need their mommy today. It can seem awfully daunting to play the dual role of mother of the year and fine-tuned baby-making machine simultaneously.

And so the pressure to have another baby blends with the stress of your current demands as a mother, wife and career woman, and you end up in the same place, but for different reasons, as your fertility sisters seeking their first child . . . angry, annoyed and exhausted!

The Angry Ovulator

Month after month, the vicious cycle continues. You experience the hope and promise of motherhood and then wake up one morning to be disappointed yet again. You maniacally chart, schedule and execute the myriad of conception counsel you've received, only to face the prospect of starting all over again. You feel like you're doing it all alone, and you're pissed.

'Til Death Do Us Part . . . Or Until I Kill You

And then it happens, like an uncontrollable nuclear reaction, a chain of events unfolds that ultimately leads to a totally destructive emotional meltdown. From this point forward, the specific event that defines your transition from a normal, rational, loving human being to an Angry Ovulator will be known as "The Incident."

Our research has shown that in most cases the events leading up to an Incident are so minor they remain undetectable to the nonovulating eye. It would be completely acceptable for a woman to go crazy if her husband walked in the door and announced he'd just lost the house on a bad bet in Vegas. Bad behavior is expected, even applauded, when a husband announces he's been cheating on his wife, secretly depleting their life savings to fund a shady habit or keeping a second wife and kids in Salt Lake City. But what about the unsuspecting husband who pours himself a glass of orange juice without asking if his wife is thirsty and receives a twenty-minute tirade about his insensitivity? He is the victim of an Angry Ovulator!

The following events leading up to and during The Incident are true. The names and identities have been withheld to protect the marriages of the innocent.

After a particularly exhausting month, one of our TTCs decided to conduct her own secret experiment in the bedroom. She had been micromanaging every detail of her procreation attempts and, quite frankly, was sick of it. Up until The Incident she had managed her husband like a business. She held status meetings, "Honey, I think I'm going to ovulate on Thursday"; sent out e-mail reminders, "The stick is almost blue; I think it's only a matter of a few more days;" and directed their bedroom activities with the precision of an air traffic controller, "If you have to travel for business tomorrow, we can get up at 5 A.M. and have sex before you go. If you catch the 8 P.M. flight home, I'll wait up, and we can do it again, so we won't actually have to miss a key day."

Then she realized her micromanaging was ridiculous and driving her crazy. What was she . . . a personal assistant? Her husband was a grown man, and he certainly had the mental capacity to remember his duties at home as well as his commitments at work. If he couldn't remember, he could simply log the information into his electronic organizer he loved so much. Her decision was made. He was on his own this month, and she couldn't wait to see what would happen.

In fairness to her husband, she couldn't go cold turkey, so she told him the day her ovulation stick announced it was time. To her surprise, the evening's events unfolded without any prodding, and the whole experience was much more pleasant for both. She really thought she was onto something with her new strategy . . . until the next day.

Her husband did not set the alarm early for a morning rendezvous, which was fine with her. She was not a morning person. But given that the stick had gone off the day before, she was due to ovulate any moment—timing was crucial. She decided to stick with her plan and see what would happen. If her husband walked in the door from work and took action, they would still be fine.

When her husband came home that night with Chinese takeout, she thought it was a good a sign. He must be thinking there was no time to spare for cooking. To her surprise, after his moo shu gai pan, he headed straight to his desk and started working on the monthly bills. Channeling all her self-control, she said nothing. When they finally went to bed and he reached over to give her a kiss and said, "Good night," she lost it.

The screaming, crying and cursing ensued, and accusations that he really didn't want children were peppered with enough four-letter words to make a truck driver blush. What was wrong with him? How many times had she told him the two days after the stick turned blue were crucial? Didn't he realize if she wasn't pregnant this month she would have to endure a series of painful tests and God knows what else? If ever her head was going to split right open, this was the day.

His Side of the Story

If he didn't know before, your husband certainly has a new level of appreciation for the stress you are under during "that time of the month." Although we do not condone his behavior, after some reflection, we can begin to understand it. As a passenger on a road trip, do you ever really pay attention to the tricky turns and side street options to beat the traffic on the freeway? No. When you know you're not going to be at the wheel, you can just kick back and enjoy the ride.

Husbands seem to have a similar attitude toward making a baby. You've been leading them through the process step-by-step, and they never expected they would have to take over the wheel. With a little warning, he probably would have done just fine, but without it, you were destined to crash.

When reflecting on the results of your first pop quiz, try to remember this—although your husband may not be on a parallel path with you on your baby-making journey, he is following closely behind, trying to keep up with your constantly changing moods and desires. Perhaps it's even a blessing you're both not living this drama 24/7. Imagine what life would be like then. Could you survive if he were constantly charting your fertile days along with you, asking for a cervical fluid report each time you came out of the ladies room? Do you really want him monitoring your daily intake of fruits and vegetables? What if he were checking in to see if your latte was decaf or if he shot you a nasty glance when you ordered a glass of wine with dinner? There is a lot of truth to the adage "ignorance is bliss." You may not want him completely clueless in the process, but be thankful he's not the sergeant at arms barking orders and reporting back with his latest findings on the benefits of yoga and acupuncture.

What Is an Angry Ovulator?

While watching one of those nature channels, a show comes on about the mating habits of the praying mantis. Normally, anything to do with an ugly bug would have you grabbing for the remote, but because it's about reproduction, you feel strangely compelled to watch. After they get through a few boring bug facts, they get to the good part. Amazingly, they capture the whole mating process on tape, and you can't believe what you're seeing. The female lures the male of choice over to her and prepares to mate. No small talk, no sexsuit and no coffee; she just rips his head off and somehow manages to conceive with what's left of him. "Lucky bug," you secretly whisper.

What exactly is an Angry Ovulator? An Angry Ovulator is a normal woman, just like you, who has been pushed too far on her quest to have a baby. She's been a good sport and even remained an optimist up until this point, but no more. She will no longer sacrifice her personal comfort for her husband's pleasure. It's time he start bearing his share of the inconvenience. When the new

Victoria's Secret catalog arrives in the mail, she takes personal offense at her husband's suggestions and swears off all lingerie for eternity. Slutty Saturday is no more. His punishment: the sexsuit is officially retired, and later that night, his old flannel boxers and the ratty Turkey Trot T-shirt make a long overdue comeback.

Bug or no bug, it looks like the male is destined to lose his head one way or another during the mating process.

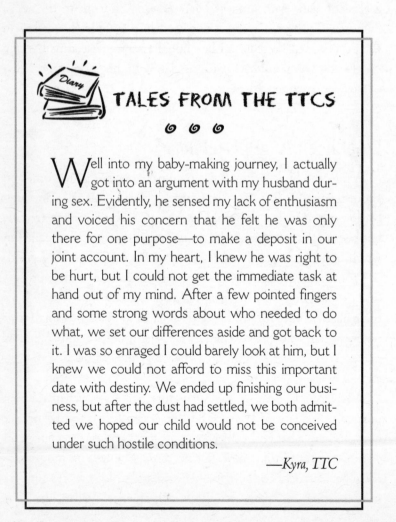

TALES FROM THE TTCS

Well into my baby-making journey, I actually got into an argument with my husband during sex. Evidently, he sensed my lack of enthusiasm and voiced his concern that he felt he was only there for one purpose—to make a deposit in our joint account. In my heart, I knew he was right to be hurt, but I could not get the immediate task at hand out of my mind. After a few pointed fingers and some strong words about who needed to do what, we set our differences aside and got back to it. I was so enraged I could barely look at him, but I knew we could not afford to miss this important date with destiny. We ended up finishing our business, but after the dust had settled, we both admitted we hoped our child would not be conceived under such hostile conditions.

—*Kyra, TTC*

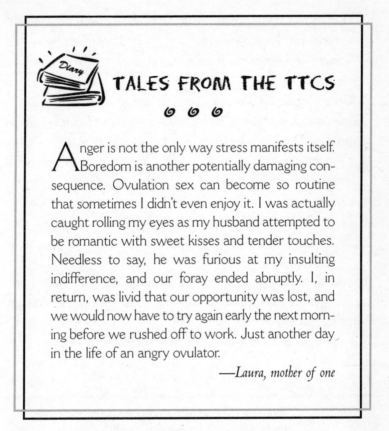

TALES FROM THE TTCS

Anger is not the only way stress manifests itself. Boredom is another potentially damaging consequence. Ovulation sex can become so routine that sometimes I didn't even enjoy it. I was actually caught rolling my eyes as my husband attempted to be romantic with sweet kisses and tender touches. Needless to say, he was furious at my insulting indifference, and our foray ended abruptly. I, in return, was livid that our opportunity was lost, and we would now have to try again early the next morning before we rushed off to work. Just another day in the life of an angry ovulator.

—*Laura, mother of one*

Could You Be an Angry Ovulator?

The first step to recovery for any bad habit is admitting you have a problem. If you cannot honestly and objectively look at your own behavior, perhaps this is the time for you to hand over the book to your husband so he can answer a few simple questions to determine your diagnosis.

1. When your husband turns up the romance and asks you to remove your tube socks, do you snap back, "No, my feet are cold!"?

2. During romantic interludes, do you secretly think to yourself, "Hurry up, I still have to _____" (fill in the blank—do laundry, make dinner, floss, finish reading the last chapter of my book, etc.)?

3. Do you wake up the morning after an angry ovulator episode full of regret for your bad behavior and try to make it up to your husband by whipping up a fancy egg dish?

4. Do you define seduction as threatening your husband with divorce if he doesn't stop what he's doing and drop his drawers that instant?

5. Has your husband accused you of having a multiple personality disorder?

If you answered "yes" to two or more of the above questions, there is a serious chance you are suffering from the Angry Ovulator syndrome. Before you program 1-800-DIVORCE into your speed dial, stop! Take it from those who have been there—there is still hope.

To:	Courtney <Courtney@conceptionchronicles.com>;
	Shelly <Shelly@conceptionchronicles.com>
From:	Patty <Patty@conceptionchronicles.com>
Subject:	**I am an Angry Ovulator!**

I've hit an all-time low. Scott got home late from work last night, again. I think he could sense how annoyed I was—so in an attempt to smooth the waters, he suggested we go out to eat.

I totally lost it. It was already 10 P.M., and we both had to get up early the next day. Normally I wouldn't care, but I AM OVULATING! I started screaming at him like a raving lunatic. He just stood there and stared at me like I had completely lost my mind (which I had).

I've got to get a grip . . . this is crazy.

Angrily yours . . .

To:	Patty <Patty@conceptionchronicles.com>
From:	Courtney <Courtney@conceptionchronicles.com>
Cc:	Shelly <Shelly@conceptionchronicles.com>
Subject:	**RE: I am an Angry Ovulator!**

Angry Ovulator??? Is that a self-diagnosis? I love it! I remember those moments; only I always thought I was just being a b*!@#.

There Is Hope for the Angry Ovulator

As if the guilt from your behavior isn't enough to contend with, now you are starting to wonder if the negative energy surging through your body during sex could impair your ability to conceive. Why would a happy, little embryo want to take up residence in such a hostile environment? You convince yourself that yes, you are once again to blame for your failed efforts, which puts even more stress on you the next month. And so the brutal cycle continues. How are you ever going to get pregnant if your overriding emotion during ovulation resembles loathing more than love?

Don't lose faith. As embarrassing as it is to admit, Angry Ovulator outbreaks are all too common. When we first came clean about our behavior, we were shocked to learn we were not alone. In hindsight, it's easy to identify the stress that tips the scales and turns you into a raving lunatic, but while you're living the moment, you can't see past the results of action or inaction. If the outcome of a month's efforts has a direct impact on your next step—for example, you will see a fertility specialist or have testing done—husbands beware. The Angry Ovulator will be out in full glory.

How do you regain control? The key to combating the angry ovulation phenomenon is recognition and avoidance. First, you must identify what triggers set you off, and then you must change your normal routine to avoid the situations that elicit this erratic (and admit it) embarrassing behavior.

For most of our TTCs, there were two key times of the month that brought out the worst in them—the three or four days before ovulation and the three or four days leading up to their next expected period. It made perfect sense. With each approaching ovulation cycle, they were overwhelmed with the sense that this could be the month—or not. The pressure to perform everything perfectly was paralyzing. Then as their period loomed over them like the green sky before a tornado, the thought of repeating it all over again the next month was too much.

When Patty realized she too had fallen into the Angry Ovulator trap, she looked at her behavior closely and realized she felt her Irish blood boiling every time she had to tell her husband, Scott, that his services were required that evening. So she decided to employ a new communications strategy. Instead of spelling out her fertile symptoms over dinner, she would simply light a lovely Yankee Gardenia candle as a sign all systems were go. Scott was briefed on the changes, and she felt the tension immediately lift knowing there was a new plan in place.

The new communications strategy was a success. Scott came home from work one night and said, "Is something burning?" After politely directing his attention to the flickering candle, nothing more needed to be said. That candle, and the many that replaced it, helped turn their bedroom barometer from tense to tranquil.

The Attraction of Distractions

Although we would rather have bamboo shoved under our fingernails than tell you to "relax" as you continually try to have a baby, we have found distracting ourselves during peak stress times to be very helpful. Try to find ways to release the negative energy. Whether it's getting a massage, taking a yoga class or reading a good trashy novel, make sure it's something that lets your mind and body escape.

One of our TTCs started taking piano lessons, as this was something she had always dreamed of doing but never found the time to actually do. Completely immersing herself into an activity so new and challenging was a great diversion from the ovulation roulette she played each month. It felt wonderful to know she was accomplishing a new goal that had absolutely nothing to do with trying to have a baby.

Another one of our TTCs rediscovered her love of tennis when the ovulation Olympics started to get to her. This allowed her to reconnect with her husband on the doubles court, and it also gave her a chance to work out her frustrations on the unsuspecting couple that paired up with them for a friendly Saturday morning match.

Whatever your distraction of choice, our most important advice for the Angry Ovulator is . . . never forget your sense of humor! Now's the time to find the humor in everything you've been through. You and your husband could certainly use a good laugh. And take it from us, once you start down the road of fertility testing, there's going to be plenty more material for your late-night comedy routine.

chapter seven

Testing, Testing . . . One, Two, Three

Wednesday   Notes

- 8 a.m. breakfast w/ boss (don't eat!)
- 9:30 a.m. blood test

Thursday   Notes

- 10:30 a.m. Ultrasound
- 3:00 p.m. Call Dr. re: blood results

Friday   Notes

- 8:00 a.m. drop off sperm sample

The first step in receiving any type of fertility treatment is to have some baseline blood work and gynecological testing done to make sure all the important parts are in place and working properly. This is where the fun begins. If you're afraid of needles, start your deep breathing exercises, because the time has come to face your fear. The good news is it really does get better. As a matter of fact, by the time you have finally completed your fertility testing, you will be so comfortable with needles, you may actually consider piercing your nipple.

The series of tests that need to be done can be a bit overwhelming, and they all start to blend together as your doctor starts rattling off the instructions for each. Some must be done before you ovulate, others after you ovulate; you must abstain from sex for three days for one test and you must have sex on the morning of another. Ask your doctor to give you printed instructions so you can keep it all straight. If not, ask him to repeat the information over and over until you are certain you'll be able to read the notes you scratched down on the back of an overdue phone bill found crumpled at the bottom of your purse.

As your doctor rattles off the information about each test and what they are for, you continually nod your head hoping to send the message, "Yes, yes, I can see how that information will be critical for making a diagnosis." When, in reality, you are fixated on just how much pain each of these tests will deliver. If you're lucky enough to have a sensitive doctor, he may sense your hesitation and prod you to voice your concerns. Don't hold back. They've heard it all before, and if creating a pain scale from 1 to 10 for each test is going to help you sleep at night, go for it.

Once your questions have been answered, you are sent on your way and told not to return until you have completed all of the required testing. The pace with which you complete these tests is entirely up to you and can vary widely from person to person.

When Patty first visited her specialist, she felt a wave of nausea when she saw what lay ahead, so she dragged her feet and remained safely tucked in her bed of denial hoping she would just get pregnant and be rescued from the torture of testing. It took her six months to face the reality and get through the basic tests. On the other hand, some of our TTCs marched into their initial consultations and within one month were back in the office mapping out their next steps. Express lane or local . . . you choose. But either way, the tests need to get done.

This Will Only Hurt for a Minute

The first stop on the fertility treatment train is blood work. Some doctors may have lab facilities in their offices, but typically these are reserved for women undergoing more serious treatment like IVF. A rookie like you will most likely be directed to an independent lab servicing the masses. Many of these labs have a fast-food mentality—walk in, take a number, sit here, blood taken, you're done . . . next! Things move along quickly, so don't expect small talk or any medical advice from your phlebotomist.

And You're Off

If you're lucky enough to be healthy, it's probably been a while since you've had your last blood test. This can be an especially trying experience for those who fear anything sharp and shiny. Of course, the initial stab of the needle hurts, especially when the nurse is rushing and doesn't give the alcohol swab time to dry, but that's not what gets the needlephobe. It's the running commentary following the piercing of the needle. The nurse starts mumbling, "Darn it, almost there, hold still, straighten your arm, darn it, keep your fist tight, almost there," all while trying to navigate the needle *inside* your arm in search of the shifty vein. You've probably seen enough episodes of *CSI* to know what's going on in there, and the visual combined with the feeling of a sharp object snaking around inside your body is enough to do in the strongest of women.

It starts slowly. The nurse's voice starts to drift far, far away and is replaced with a subtle and familiar buzz. You're confident you can will yourself to stay conscious, so you start thinking happy thoughts: sunny beach, favorite dessert, winning tonight's Powerball drawing. Too late. The room starts to blur, and a gray haze provides a backdrop for a sea of twinkling stars. You try to calmly announce you're starting to feel a little dizzy, but it's out of your control—you've already hit the floor. You are utterly humiliated when you regain consciousness to a room full of people scrambling to bring in a portable cot. "It's okay, it's okay," you reassure them. "It happens all the time."

Their response certainly wasn't what they learned during compassion class at nursing school, "If you knew you were going to faint, you should have said something. We would have taken your blood with you lying down." How do you explain that since you're a grown adult, you were hoping this experience would be slightly better than your second-grade tonsillectomy, which ended with you being held down by two nurses as the third rammed a needle the size of a screwdriver into your buttocks. Clearly you have no defense; after all, you're the one on the floor. You have no choice but to acquiesce. "Yes, of course, I will definitely wait for the cot the next time," you weakly reply.

When you are confident you can stand long enough to make the sprint from the office directly to your car, you pull yourself together as best you can and make a run for it. "See you next week," you toss out perkily as you grab for the door.

To:	Courtney <Courtney@conceptionchronicles.com>;
	Shelly <Shelly@conceptionchronicles.com>
From:	Patty <Patty@conceptionchronicles.com>
Subject:	**Irony**

Don't you think it's ironic my veins are the only part of my body that could be considered unusually small!

To:	Patty <Patty@conceptionchronicles.com>
From:	Courtney <Courtney@conceptionchronicles.com>
Cc:	Shelly <Shelly@conceptionchronicles.com>
Subject:	**RE: Irony**

That's not true . . . your boobs are unusually small too!

Am I Normal?

Your doctor will request blood work on several different days for baseline testing. Although each doctor may vary slightly in the tests they perform, the blood test on day three of your cycle is pretty standard. Before we get to the blood work, let's review how you actually count the days of your menstrual cycle. The first day of your cycle is the day you have a full flow of red blood. Yuck. We know it's descriptive, but this will save you many calls to the doctor's office. Many women experience light spotting, which turns to full flow a day or two later. The actual transition from spotting to flow may not be obvious, so a general rule of thumb is the day you need to wear protection is considered day one. Here's a quick glimpse at the baseline blood tests and the days they are performed:

Hormone	Cycle Day of Test	What It Means
Follicle Stimulating Hormone (FSH)	Day 3	FSH is used as a gauge of ovarian reserve. A day-three FSH of less than 10mIU/ml is preferred. An elevated number can be a sign of diminished ovarian reserve.
Estrodial (estrogen)	Day 3	A woman's cycle starts off with relatively low levels of estrogen, which continue to rise as she approaches ovulation. When it reaches a high enough level, the body is triggered to begin ovulation. Abnormally high levels on day three may indicate a cyst or diminished ovarian reserve. Normal results on day three are between 10 and 60pg/ml.
Luteinizing Hormone (LH)	Day 3	A normal level is generally less than 7mIU/ml.

Hormone	Cycle Day of Test	What It Means
Luteinizing Hormone (LH)	Surge day	LH is the checkered flag that starts the ovulation race. Once the estrogen signals the body it's time to ovulate, the large quantity of LH released literally causes the egg to burst out of the follicle. Levels should rise to more than 20mIU/ml.
Progesterone	Day 3	A day-three test should show a low level of less than 1.5ng/ml.
Progesterone	Post ovulation Days 22–24	A progesterone test is done to confirm ovulation. Once a woman ovulates, the empty follicle left behind produces proges-terone. A level over 10ng/ml indicates ovulation occurred.

Disclaimer: Values presented are an average, and labs have varying standards to which they adhere.

The Vaginal Ultrasound: Hello Up There!

Some doctors prefer to use a vaginal ultrasound to get an up close and personal look at the inner workings of all things female. Our impression of an ultrasound before we actually had one was what we had always seen on television. We expected the nurse to squirt some gooey jelly on our stomachs and then slide a metal paddle across our bellies to reveal the fine workings of our feminine organs. Yes, that is the procedure for an *abdominal* ultrasound, but apparently the PG-13 version is saved for women who are already pregnant.

For those of us still trying to have a baby, they need to get an insider's view. The vaginal ultrasound machine has a "wand," which is inserted into your vagina and can be moved around to get a clear view of your ovaries and uterus. When you first glance at the ultrasound machine, you may be slightly intimidated by all of the wires, buttons and switches. You may not even notice the wand initially—at least, not until the nurse comes in, unwraps a condom and slides it over the giant plastic probe. We're not talking a wand the size of a tampon; we're talking the equivalent of a Six Flags giant souvenir pencil whose sole purpose was to show off your summer vacation to your fourth-grade class because it was clearly too big for writing. Before you have a chance to ask where that thing is going, it's too late—you're already deflowered.

Shocking . . . yes. Painful . . . no. Of course, it does make a difference who's at the controls. If you happen to be the last appointment of the day, look out. This is not a test you want to rush. But seriously, even if you have Speedy Gonzalez racing from your left ovary to your right, it really doesn't hurt. The worst we can say is it's a bit uncomfortable.

Once you get past the initial shock and awkwardness of the first ultrasound, you may be surprised when you actually start looking forward to the test as it becomes a routine part of fertility treatment. Ovulation sticks are child's play in comparison to the ultrasound. It really is amazing. You can literally look inside your ovaries and see how many follicles you have, how they are growing and, ultimately, exactly when you ovulate. If only you could get one of these machines at home, the ovulation predictor sticks would be history. You've decided if you're not pregnant by Christmas, the G.E. Logic 400 Proseries ultrasound machine is going to be at the top of your wish list.

READER/CUSTOMER CARE SURVEY

We care about your opinions! Please take a moment to fill out our online Reader Survey at **http://survey.hcibooks.com.**
As a **"THANK YOU"** you will receive a **VALUABLE INSTANT COUPON** towards future book purchases
as well as a **SPECIAL GIFT** available only online! Or, you may mail this card back to us.

(PLEASE PRINT IN ALL CAPS)

First Name _____ MI. _____ Last Name _____

Address _____ City _____

State _____ Zip _____ Email _____

1. Gender
☐ Female   ☐ Male

2. Age
☐ 8 or younger   ☐ 13-16
☐ 9-12   ☐ 21-30
☐ 17-20
☐ 31+

3. Did you receive this book as a gift?
☐ Yes   ☐ No

4. Annual Household Income
☐ under $25,000
☐ $25,000 - $34,999
☐ $35,000 - $49,999
☐ $50,000 - $74,999
☐ over $75,000

5. What are the ages of the children living in your house?
☐ 0 - 14   ☐ 15+

6. Marital Status
☐ Single
☐ Married
☐ Divorced
☐ Widowed

7. How did you find out about the book?
(please choose one)
☐ Recommendation
☐ Store Display
☐ Online
☐ Catalog/Mailing
☐ Interview/Review

8. Where do you usually buy books?
(please choose one)
☐ Bookstore
☐ Online
☐ Book Club/Mail Order
☐ Price Club (Sam's Club, Costco's, etc.)
☐ Retail Store (Target, Wal-Mart, etc.)

9. What subject do you enjoy reading about the most?
(please choose one)
☐ Parenting/Family
☐ Relationships
☐ Recovery/Addictions
☐ Health/Nutrition
☐ Christianity
☐ Spirituality/Inspiration
☐ Business Self-help
☐ Women's Issues
☐ Sports

10. What attracts you most to a book?
(please choose one)
☐ Title
☐ Cover Design
☐ Author
☐ Content

TAPE IN MIDDLE; DO NOT STAPLE

BUSINESS REPLY MAIL
FIRST-CLASS MAIL   PERMIT NO 45   DEERFIELD BEACH, FL

POSTAGE WILL BE PAID BY ADDRESSEE

Health Communications, Inc.
3201 SW 15th Street
Deerfield Beach FL 33442-9875

FOLD HERE

Comments

The Semen Analysis: Is This Gun Loaded?

Finally, your husband, who's been on deck for months, is up to bat. Although you secretly feel some annoyance that his test involves cruising porn and doing something he's been doing for pleasure since high school, you are also relieved the fertility microscope is pointed at someone other than you.

The semen analysis can be much trickier than you originally thought. First, there are the logistics. Typically, the patient is asked to abstain from sexual relations for at least three but no longer than five days before having the test. Apparently, too much or too little sex can impact the quality of the sperm. After weeks of monotonous sex on demand, a medical prescription for guilt-free abstinence is an unexpected bonus. Of course, you don't want to risk any opportunity to conceive, so you must carefully schedule this test when you are certain you are well past ovulation.

The next hurdle is the collection. The sample must arrive at the lab within forty-five to sixty minutes from the time of ejaculation, and it must be protected from exposure to heat or cold while being transported. If you happen to live close by the recommended lab, your husband will be sent home with a specimen cup and a list of dos and don'ts when medically masturbating. However, if there's no way you can make it to the lab within an hour, it may be necessary for your husband to produce his sample on site. Short of being diagnosed with a terminal illness, this is the worst possible news a man can hear. Fear not. It shouldn't be too hard to find another lab or hospital close to your home. Just place a quick call to your doctor to be certain the lab's standards are up to par. You don't want to learn two months later that the garage next door offering "$29.99 lube and oil changes" was actually operated by the same people who were analyzing the quality of your husband's sperm.

Once you have the location confirmed, it's time to produce the goods. While your husband may complain the instruction sheet is a buzz kill, we take much greater pity on the fathers of the world who are expected to produce a sample while their three-year-old bangs on the bathroom door screaming, "Daddy, I need to use the potty."

After all you've been through with the magic ultrasound wand, it will be hard to work up some sincere sympathy when your husband proudly emerges from the bathroom and displays his sample exclaiming, "Wow, that was really hard." Of course, if the complaining persists without garnering results, you can always volunteer to help things along. If you aren't comfortable, or quite frankly not interested, there's always the Playboy channel. Tell your husband you're giving him a free pass to enjoy his new membership to www.bigboobs.com while he can.

Remember, the clock starts ticking once the gun is fired, so you must immediately race to the lab. If you have the pleasure of dropping off the sample, start the two-man relay by tucking the container into your bra to keep it nice and toasty for the drive. Next, you must prepare yourself for the inevitable humiliation to follow. While the receptionist maintains a normal speaking voice for those who are in for their annual flu shot, her volume and projection rival a Broadway diva when she announces they are ready to accept the SEMEN SAMPLE! So much for the brown paper bag—the jig is up; you must try to maintain some level of dignity as you hand over the magical elixir.

TALES FROM THE TTCS

I received a prescription for a semen analysis from my doctor. The form detailed the requested analysis on one side and all the participating labs, along with their hours of operation, on the back. My husband and I were relieved to find a lab just a few miles from our house, and we were even happier when we noticed the lab opened at 6 A.M. How convenient! We wouldn't even be late for work. So a few days later, we arrived promptly at 6 A.M. with our sample, only to be greeted by a giggling receptionist who informed us the lab technicians didn't arrive until 10 A.M., so the sample would be unusable. We were sent home and told to try again after abstaining for another three days. After setting up and confirming our next appointment, we arrived with brown bag in tow. When we mentioned to a new receptionist this was our second attempt, she quickly said, "Oh, you're the 6 A.M. couple," and started to laugh as she began filling out the paperwork. It was nice to know our humiliating experience had provided some good water-cooler gossip.

—Lucy, mother of one

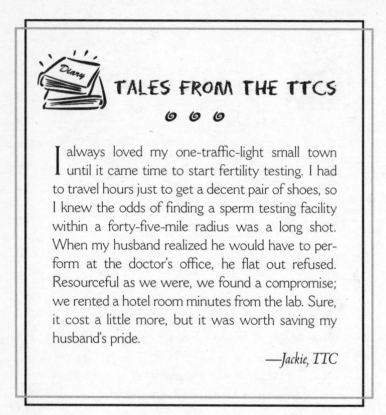

TALES FROM THE TTCS

I always loved my one-traffic-light small town until it came time to start fertility testing. I had to travel hours just to get a decent pair of shoes, so I knew the odds of finding a sperm testing facility within a forty-five-mile radius was a long shot. When my husband realized he would have to perform at the doctor's office, he flat out refused. Resourceful as we were, we found a compromise; we rented a hotel room minutes from the lab. Sure, it cost a little more, but it was worth saving my husband's pride.

—*Jackie, TTC*

Is He Normal?

The purpose of the semen analysis is to check the quantity and quality of sperm in the ejaculate. Roughly a third of all infertility cases are a result of male factors, so this simple test is a logical step in your initial workup. Although the standards for a quality semen analysis may vary a bit among doctors, the World Health Organization has defined the standard for a quality semen sample as having a volume level of 40 million or more sperm per ejaculate—60 percent or more should be moving, and at least 30 percent should be normally shaped. If your husband happens to exceed the normal standards, prepare yourself for months of gloating. He's so proud of his virility you're certain he has added his sperm count to his résumé right along with his academic honors and community service awards.

Of course, age does play a role in the reproductive game, regardless of the player. So even if your man still has his hair, can bench press a small elephant and runs a mile in under six minutes, if he's inching toward forty, his sperm count may show it.

Don't panic if the initial results come back with questionable findings. Sperm production often varies from sample to sample, so your doctor will most likely order another test before drawing any conclusions. Once your doctor has all the information, he will factor in your husband's age and announce his verdict. Even if you do end up facing some male fertility issues, all hope is not lost. There are plenty of treatments available to overcome many problems associated with low sperm count or poor motility.

Taking It Up a Notch

The timing and need for the next series of tests will be determined based on the results of the initial testing and your doctor's desire for a second home in Maui. While each doctor's opinion may vary slightly on what tests need to be done before making a diagnosis, the Postcoital Test and the Hysterosalpingogram (HSG) are pretty standard. If you thought the semen analysis was an embarrassing proposition, you ain't seen nothing yet!

The Postcoital Test: The New Walk of Shame

Yes . . . the name says it all. No need for your doctor to spell this one out. You have a basic idea of what you're in for the minute he utters the words. The purpose of the postcoital test is to take a look at your cervical fluid and how your husband's sperm behaves in that fluid to see if things are moving along as swimmingly as they should. Although rarely discussed at parties, cervical fluid is the unsung hero of the reproductive process. Like your favorite bouncer at a hot new club, when there's good-quality cervical fluid at the door, sperm are ushered along to the VIP area with little effort. Without it, they're stopped dead in their tracks and left standing out in the cold only to dream of what lies beyond the red velvet rope.

The postcoital test must be done around the time you ovulate, so once again it's time to break out the supersize box of ovulation sticks. You will be instructed to call the doctor's office the day you see the LH surge. Your doctor will then try to cram your test into his next day's already packed schedule, which means you will either be arriving at the crack of dawn or waiting in the reception area for at least an hour. He will specify what time you should have sex that evening; typically it's anywhere from six to twelve hours before the test. You'll also be given detailed instructions on the rules and regulations of postcoital test sex. The instruction sheet is reminiscent of the advice your mother would give before heading off to spring break, "Don't get a room on the first floor of the hotel. Don't go to bars. Don't sit in the sun too long. Don't talk to strangers. Don't accept a ride from anyone other than a professional taxi company . . . and have a good time!"

As you can imagine, the pressure to perform for the postcoital test makes sex on demand look like a honeymoon special. Knowing someone will be snooping around "down there" the next morning dampens the mood almost as much as you reading the instructions to your husband for the evening's activities. Careful not to miss a single detail, you whip out the postcoital information sheet and begin, "We will be having sex at 11:30 P.M. Use of a lubricant of any kind is forbidden; this includes K-Y Jelly, Vaseline, baby oil, and so on. Following intercourse, I'll remain lying down for thirty minutes. You are responsible for the postcoital snack and beverage service. I may shower in the morning, but I cannot bathe or douche." You close your presentation with, "Got it, honey? Okay, let's get started."

What Happens When the Equipment Fails?

In fine print at the bottom of the postcoital test instruction sheet, there is an innocent line about many couples not being able to perform under the pressure of the situation. If this happens, it states, you are to call the office in the morning and reschedule. You breeze past this information—up until this point, even sex under duress, while it may not have been particularly earthmoving for either of you, has never been a problem. You know there have been several times when your husband really wasn't in the mood, but the calendar ruled, and even under the most sleep-deprived, tense situations, it has always worked out. Worst case scenario, you broke out the big guns. We're not going to go into details, but you girls know exactly what we're talking about.

Then out of the blue it happens. Even with the dirtiest of talk, the equipment simply fails. Great. Although this may be a first, you must try to understand the enormity of the situation. Culturally, men have been raised to closely identify with their sexuality. In many ways, it defines them. It's a sign of their manhood . . . the strut factor. That's why right now there are young men across America exaggerating the outcome of last night's uneventful date. It's the root of the male ego and the inspiration for the greatest song on the Grease soundtrack, "Summer Lovin'."

Just like you never thought you would have a hard time conceiving, your husband never imagined he wouldn't be "man enough" to get you pregnant. The postcoital test challenges the very essence of his manhood. Of course, this is what he's thinking . . . not you.

And so the colossal consequences race through his mind, which in turn sends a shut-down message to his libido, which makes him further question his manhood, and round and round he goes until his world crashes, and there's no hope for recovery. Time to admit defeat. The postcoital test needs to be rescheduled.

Of course, you feel bad for your husband, but you feel even worse for yourself as you pick up the phone to call the doctor's office the next morning. After apologizing for making everyone come in early for the test that wouldn't happen, you quietly thank the nurse for understanding and hang up the phone. You're certain everyone in the office is talking about you and your failed attempts in the bedroom. Just when you convince yourself these are trained medical professionals, and you're being paranoid, your doctor greets you at your next appointment with, "So he has trouble performing under pressure." You are so insulted you immediately come to your husband's defense and explain this is the first time anything like this has ever happened and start rattling off a list of reasons for his subpar performance: he had a fever, he just finished running a marathon, we had sex the twelve prior consecutive days, and so on. You're sure it was an isolated incident. With the look of a teacher who's heard every excuse in the book, he dismissively says, "Fine, we'll try again next month."

RELATIONSHIP RESCUE

The endless poking and prodding, along with all the embarrassing situations, can leave even the strongest of marriages a bit rickety. If you find this to be the case, then it's probably time to resuscitate your relationship. We found that this doesn't take much energy, and simple things go a long way. It's making the effort that really counts. We know you've heard it countless times before—that's right, the highly touted "Date

Night." We snickered at the thought that a scheduled night out each week with our husbands would actually make a difference, but it works. There is one prerequisite: no fertility discussions allowed! You can talk about anything—what to plant in the garden this spring, your plans to repave the driveway or the fact that the sprinklers aren't working the way they should. But whatever you do, give yourselves a much-needed break from talking about the countless tests you've endured and speculating on their meaning.

On the contrary, you should also set aside one night a week to thoroughly discuss every detail of your fertility regime. It's the antidate night—it's "Debate Night." You know by now it's not easy to talk about your fertility issues when emotions are running high. And trying to discuss potential treatment options on the ten-minute drive back to work after a doctor's appointment has probably led to some less-than-productive (or healthy) exchanges. Many of our TTCs agree that it's much easier to talk about how they're feeling after they've had time to digest the information and organize their thoughts.

There are a couple of simple rules to be followed on Debate Night. It's important to let your husband speak, and try to refrain from responding to every single comment or train of thought he might have. Really listen to what he is saying before you respond. You both have strong feelings and opinions surrounding the issues, and you need to give each other the freedom to say what's on your mind and in your heart. The best part of setting time aside is knowing you'll both have an opportunity to say everything you want and need to say and that your concerns will be heard.

The Hysterosalpingogram (HSG):
Pronunciation Not a Prerequisite

Like Big Foot, the Loch Ness Monster and the Bermuda Triangle, in the fertility world nothing conjures up stories of fear like the hysterosalpingogram. (Don't worry if you can't pronounce it; neither can we.) The HSG, for those of us who stumble on seven-syllable words, is basically an x-ray image of the uterus and fallopian tubes. Before being photographed, the uterus is filled with dye, which should overflow into the fallopian tubes if there are no blockages. The dye provides contrast, defining the organs, and allows the x-rays to be more easily read. The purpose of this test is to get a detailed look at the path a sperm must take in order to achieve pregnancy and make sure there are no unexpected roadblocks along the way.

Unfortunately, to capture these images, you must endure a somewhat invasive and uncomfortable procedure. Essentially, the equivalent of a garden hose is thread through your vagina into your cervix. The doctor then gives the thumbs up sign to his assistant, and dye begins shooting out of the hose at a shocking velocity, filling your uterus. The sensation is hard to explain, but the closest we can get to describing it is the reverse feeling of relief when you really, really, really have to go to the bathroom. In this case, you can actually feel the liquid filling your uterus, along with a pressure that screams, "I've got to pee."

Once you are all juiced up, your doctor may ask you to roll from side to side to see if the dye freely flows into both of the fallopian tubes. All throughout this process the cameras are rolling and capturing the details of your uterine environment. Before you get off the table, your doctor should be able to tell you if everything looks normal as well as if there are any fibroid tumors or polyps infringing on your uterine cavity. If there are, they may be creating a problem when the embryo tries to nestle in for the nine-month nap.

Before you know it, the test is over, and the nurse is handing you a sample of what you thought had long been extinct . . . a four-inch-thick Modess Maxi Pad, complete with six-inch straps on either side. Apparently these pads are still in circulation, and you are the lucky recipient of the excess inventory, sans the belt. You now have a whole new obsession. Can anyone see the encyclopedia in my panties? Note to self: for all future testing that requires organs to be filled with fluid, avoid tight-fitting pants, wear skirt and B.Y.O.M.—bring your own streamlined maxipad for discreet protection.

We're certainly not discounting the potential painfulness of this test. But before we actually had the test ourselves, we had only heard the urban legends of pain and anguish around the HSG. Our doctors and friends told us to take pain medication *before* the test. By the time our appointments finally arrived, we had ourselves so worked up we nearly fainted just thinking about it. Like most things, however, the hype was far worse than the reality.

We were lucky we didn't have any blockages, which, according to some of our TTCs, can cause additional pain. So for us, the test really wasn't that bad. In fact, thinking back, if we had the choice between an HSG and an armpit wax at Coco Nails, the HSG would win every time.

One TTC who went in for an HSG said that although the test was not nearly as painful as she expected, it certainly was eventful. As she lay naked on an examining table with nothing but a sheet of tissue paper between her and a very high-tech x-ray machine, she realized there was quite an audience for her uterine debut. Her doctor and an assistant were in the room to perform the procedure, and a technician was tucked away in a glass booth, where he would be operating the x-ray equipment throughout the test.

The procedure got off to a rough start as the doctor fumbled while trying to insert the tube into her cervix. This certainly wasn't pleasant, but it was over quickly. Before she could catch her breath, the doctor instructed the assistant to start the flow of dye. What happened next is a bit of a blur. Our TTC could feel her uterus filling, and then, all of a sudden, dye was spraying everywhere. The room took on the intensity of an unscripted episode of *E.R.* The Wizard of Oz technician was heard screaming over the intercom system for the doctor to shift the tube to the right. The doctor completely ignored him and forged ahead through the liquid storm of medical-grade x-ray dye. At one point, TTC heard the doctor yell something about a "TUMOR"; the doctor then barked a series of commands that had her flipping from left to right, like a fish out of water.

As she lay there naked in complete shock trying to process the fact that she must have cancer, she struggled to regain her composure. After she got dressed, she looked around for her doctor, desperate to learn more about her condition. Too late. Her doctor was long gone—she had already moved on to ruin someone else's life. As it turned out, our TTC did not have cancer, and her very common "fibroid" tumor would not play a role in her attempts to conceive—and neither would her current doctor. She found a new one the very next day.

Ch . . . Ch . . . Changes

Although there may never be a convenient time to change doctors, if you're not comfortable with your physician's competency or bedside manner after the initial round of testing, it's probably a good time to start the search again. Some doctors may insist on repeating some of the tests you've already done, but many will be happy to simply review the x-rays or lab results. Going back to the starting block and taking the tests over can be a hard pill to swallow. You may initially try to talk yourself into sticking with your current doctor just to keep the ball moving even though you know it's not the right fit. Take it from us; one small step back in your treatment could be a giant step forward for your mental health and your ultimate success. In the grand scheme of things, an extra month or two will be well worth the sacrifice if you end up finding a doctor who truly understands your desire to have a baby and all the frustrations that go along with it when you just can't seem to get there.

To: Shelly <Shelly@conceptionchronicles.com>;
      Courtney <Courtney@conceptionchronicles.com>
From: Patty <Patty@conceptionchronicles.com>
Subject: **That's it!**

I need to find a new doctor. I've never felt comfortable with mine, but today's appointment took the cake. She spent the first ten minutes of my "consultation" complaining about how expensive it is to send her two children to Ivy League schools. By the time we finally got around to me, she barely had time to rush through my test results before doing the exam (which I swear took less than five minutes).

Before I could blurt out a question, she was out the door, leaving me with my feet sky high in the stirrups. I've totally had it. Even if she doesn't give a crap, the least she could do is fake it. But I dread the thought of starting this process all over. What if I switch doctors and have to go through all these tests again?

To: Patty <Patty@conceptionchronicles.com>
From: Shelly <Shelly@conceptionchronicles.com>
Cc: Courtney <Courtney@conceptionchronicles.com>
Subject: **RE: That's it!**

Sounds like it's time to move on—even if you have to do some of the tests over again, at least you know what to expect. This is definitely a time when bedside manner counts. Take the time to find someone you are comfortable with and trust. Don't worry; everything happens for a reason.

There's No Room for Modesty at the Infertility Inn

Remember the old days when you would try in vain to cover yourself with the twelve inch by twenty-four inch paper napkin the nurse handed you in the changing area. As if to make it seem possible, the nurse would always say, "Please remove everything and put on the dressing gown." Was she serious? Unless you were an origami expert, there was no way it would even cover the good parts.

No one was happier than you when the doctor upgraded to the slightly more fashionable fertility separates. Now you were handed two pieces when you walked into the examining room—a vest and a skirt, or so it said on the package. In reality, it was just another square of tracing paper with three holes of equal size cut at awkward angles. You assume one hole is for your head and the other two are for your arms, but there are literally hundreds of configurations that all work, each exposing various body parts along the way.

After countless doctor appointments and fertility tests, your modesty becomes a distant relative, familiar, but certainly not top of mind. The next time the nurse hands you the latest in paper ready-to-wear, you don't even bother to put it on. You simply toss it over your arm like a beach towel and hop on the table. You'll keep it handy in case there's a fire, but barring any emergencies, you are at one with your naked self.

Sabbatical Recommended for Graduate-Level Testing

For those of you with A+ organs, there's really no reason to read any further. For you, the cyclone of testing has come to a complete stop. Feel free to unbuckle your seatbelt and exit the ride in an orderly fashion.

But for those of you who may have had some questionable results or who continue to show symptoms indicating things may be a bit off-kilter, your doctor may want to take an even closer look. Closer than the magic ultrasound wand? Yes, closer than the magic ultrasound wand.

Laparoscopy: Front Row Seats

There is good news and bad news with the laparoscopy. The good news is, you will be out cold under general anesthesia during the procedure and won't remember a thing when you finally wake up in recovery. The bad news is, your belly button's sole purpose is no longer to provide a marker for acceptability when purchasing low-ride jeans. Your belly button is now viewed as a portal to the inner you, and sharp scary things are going to be forcing their way through it to get a good look at what's happening under the hood. The purpose of this surgical procedure is to look at your organs from a perspective that is not visible with an ultrasound.

You should receive a packet of information in advance outlining the procedure and what you need to do to prepare for the surgery. Typically, you are not allowed to eat or drink anything after midnight, but there's also a warning about dehydration. At 11:45 P.M. the night before your operation, you should be slurping down a Super Big Gulp of water.

On the day of your laparoscopy, you will be told to arrive at the hospital a few hours before the actual procedure. All the pre-op instructions will make it sound like this time is necessary for all the prep required before surgery; in reality, they really just want the extra hours to make sure your insurance is up to date and someone will be paying the bill.

Once all the paperwork is complete, you are issued the standard hospital ID bracelet. You are then led into a room where a nurse takes your blood pressure, collects a urine sample and starts an IV. Next, you are wheeled to the operating room, which will undoubtedly have giant white lights and a medical staff of people looking adequately germ-free donning operating masks, hair nets and rubber gloves.

Your new best friend, the anesthesiologist, arrives and asks you some stupid question about your favorite vacation. Before you can answer, you are lulled off to a deep, wonderful sleep. When Patty had her laparoscopy, her greatest fear was she would be paralyzed from the medication, unable to cry out for help but still able to feel the pain. This seed had been planted in her head from the many horror stories her nurse friend had told over the years. She was fine, and you will be too. The guys with the drugs know what they're doing.

Your doctor will make an incision in your belly button and one or two below your bikini line. He inserts a lighted telescope into the abdominal cavity and inflates the space with gas so he can move around more easily. He will insert a laser through the bikini line incision, which will be used to remove any endometriosis or scar tissue. If you do have endometriosis or scar tissue, it can prevent the organs from moving freely and inhibit your ability to get pregnant. We've known several TTCs who got pregnant just months after having a laparoscopy.

After the procedure, you're rolled back to recovery, left to rest until the anesthesia wears off and then moved back to a standard room where you get to watch bad daytime TV. The laparoscopy is usually done on an outpatient basis, so as soon as you can slug back some 7-Up and eat a piece of dry toast, the staff will grab your coat and show you to the door.

Hysteroscopy: While You're in There

While you're under for the laparoscopy, your doctor may choose to perform a hysteroscopy. This can also be done in the doctor's office, but as far as we're concerned, the more testing that can be done when unconscious, the better. This test is very similar to the HSG, but in this case, the cavity is distended with gas and a microscope is inserted through the cervix, into the uterus and up to the fallopian tubes. This allows doctors to detect small polyps or fibroid tumors that may have been invisible in the HSG. If your doctor feels these tumors are a problem, he may remove them during the procedure. If you are having the procedure done in his office, you may need to schedule outpatient surgery.

To: Courtney <Courtney@conceptionchronicles.com>;
          Shelly <Shelly@conceptionchronicles.com>
From: Patty <Patty@conceptionchronicles.com>
Subject: **Feed a cold, starve a laparoscopy**

My mom came up to help out for a few days after my laparoscopy. Scott's been working so much, I knew he couldn't take more than a day off. It was so sweet; my mom made a huge pot of my favorite soup. But I couldn't really eat because my stomach was upset—I just had a small cup and hit the bed.

A nap and a couple of painkillers later, I was feeling much better and ready to dive into a big bowl. Too late. Scott had eaten it all for dinner . . . literally every drop.

To:	Patty <Patty@conceptionchronicles.com>
From:	Shelly <Shelly@conceptionchronicles.com>
Cc:	Courtney <Courtney@conceptionchronicles.com>
Subject:	**RE: Feed a cold, starve a laparoscopy**

Moron.

To:	Patty <Patty@conceptionchronicles.com>
From:	Courtney <Courtney@conceptionchronicles.com>
Cc:	Shelly <Shelly@conceptionchronicles.com>
Subject:	**RE: RE: Feed a cold, starve a laparoscopy**

Idiot.

That's a Wrap

Of course, there are countless tests that can be performed to identify reproductive problems, but the ones listed here are the basics. Once you have completed all the testing, your doctor should have enough information to make a preliminary diagnosis and recommend a treatment plan. Pat yourself on the back; you've made it this far. Keep your eye on the prize—it's on to the next step.

chapter eight

The Psychotic Supplement

Sunday   Notes

- Drugstore:
  - toothpaste
  - detergent
  - Clomid

Monday   Notes   Tuesday   Notes

You've been nervously anticipating the results of your tests and are cautiously relieved to once again be sitting in your doctor's office waiting to hear your diagnosis. You'll finally have the answers to your questions and will be able to move forward with a treatment plan. Maybe . . . maybe not. Your doctor may be able to give you a clear diagnosis of your fertility issues; if this is the case, believe it or not, you should consider yourself lucky. However, for many couples, the answer they receive after their initial testing can be even more frustrating than the many months that have passed while they've unsuccessfully tried to get pregnant. Your doctor's words, "Everything looks good," are a bit misleading upon first hearing them. Just when you finish letting out a deep sigh of relief, he follows up with, "You have what we call unexplained infertility." Sadly, for one-third of all fertility patients, their specialists cannot find an explanation for the couples' inability to conceive.

Your doctor continues to say that while he can give you no specific diagnosis right now, the early steps of treatment are pretty standard anyway—common in fact. You're thinking, "If I were shopping for a T-shirt, this one-size-fits-all approach would be fine, but we're talking about ME and MY chances of having a baby." Your mind flashes back to a conversation you had a few months ago with a girlfriend. She asked how things were going with your attempts, and you answered your customary, "Fine. We're still trying." Her response shocked you: "If you've been trying this long without any luck, there's obviously something wrong." At the time, you could not—would not—agree with her. And now, after finally admitting there might be a problem, you are being delivered the ultimate bad news. Yes, there's something wrong. We just don't know what it is.

You snap back to the present and return to information-gathering mode. You start asking questions about your next steps—precisely what the treatment is and when you'll start. The doctor rattles off answers to each of your questions and ends your appointment by handing you a prescription: clomiphene citrate. Of course, Clomid. The fertility wonder drug. As you leave the office, you rack your brain trying to remember everyone you know who ever took it.

The minute you get home, you call your mom to fill her in on all of your good news. No, they don't have a diagnosis, and even better, you will be taking fertility drugs that will increase your chances of giving birth to multiples. You prepare her with the news that her Florida time-share may soon be on the block to help with the twins' college fund.

C'mon, Everybody's Doing It

If you loosely toss out to your inner circle of friends that you are considering taking Clomid, we're certain several will chime in with their own personal stories or secondhand narratives of those who have taken the magic pill. It seems everyone knows someone who has taken Clomid at one point in her reproductive life. You've heard countless stories about women who take it, and the next thing you know, they're pregnant with twins. Your mom even confirmed that your Aunt Peggy, after years of failed attempts, did indeed take Clomid to get pregnant with your cousin Mary. The fact is, Clomid has been circulating in the fertility world for years, and it's usually the first recommended treatment from doctors when trying to get pregnant on your own isn't working.

Still, the decision to begin Clomid is often not easy, and you may experience one of two common reactions when you consider taking it. You may think back to your initial consultation with your doctor where he laid out the three steps of fertility treatment—1. Clomid. 2. Injectable drugs. 3. In vitro fertilization. You immediately think, "Oh my God, I am two steps away from having a test-tube baby!" On the other hand, you may be like many other women who see taking Clomid as a relatively simple first step. If all they need to do to get pregnant is take a pill, then sign 'em up.

To further complicate matters, for the six to fifteen million who experience "secondary infertility" (or trouble conceiving a second child), the decision to take fertility medication can be even more difficult. If you've successfully conceived and delivered a child without fertility assistance, the choice to begin treatment can be complex. You may wrestle with the fact that you were able to conceive on your own just a few years earlier, so what has changed? Doesn't the body retain crucial baby-making information? Admitting you need help is an unwelcome decision. Taking a pill is the easy part. Swallowing your infertility issues is agonizing.

One Small Step in Treatment, One Giant Step Toward Motherhood

Whether you struggle with your decision to take Clomid or come to it rather easily, beginning fertility treatment can raise the question, "What lies ahead?" Once these hormones are in your system, will you ever really know where nature ends and science begins? Let's face it, you've gone au natural this far, and you're still not pregnant. You're getting help from doctors who know what they're doing, and it's time to put your trust in the treatment process. Look at it positively. You're moving forward, not backward, and taking this first step is getting you closer to motherhood.

Even after you've consciously made the choice to begin your Clomid treatment, you may still seek confirmation you are doing the right thing, even from the most unusual sources. One of our TTCs who was struggling for number two began taking advice from random strangers, desperate to reinforce her decision. Sitting at the park one day while her two-year-old played nearby, she began divulging her fertility woes to a woman who had unwittingly asked if she had any other children. It seems the innocent bystander was quite familiar with Clomid and its reported benefits and suggested our TTC give it a try because she knew many women who had been successful with it. Our TTC was clearly looking for a sign—any sign—that she should try Clomid. Maybe it was the hot sun going to her head, or she just wanted to hear from another woman she was making the right decision. Nevertheless, our TTC filled her prescription the next day.

All Aboard!

After your minifocus groups are complete, you conclude Clomid is about as common as taking aspirin when embarking on the early stages of fertility treatment. You understand Clomid will help you ovulate if you're not already doing so or regulate your cycle so you produce multiple eggs, which will inevitably increase your odds of pregnancy.

Just like the kick-start you feel when going back to the gym after a long sabbatical, this may be just what your female organs need to get them going again. When you mention to your husband that you will begin taking Clomid this month, he says, "Fine by me. What is it?" He surprises you with his curiosity, and as you begin to reply, you quickly realize you really don't know all that much about it. It's back to Google to find out exactly what this drug is and what havoc it will wreak on your body and your brain.

Good Things Come in Small Packages

As you wait for your computer to boot up, you try to evoke bits and pieces of the conversation you had with your doctor when he initially explained Clomid and its benefits. He gave you the general description, "It will *help* you ovulate," and then pointed to a picture of his wife and two beautiful boys telling you that they are Clomid twins. Cute. At the time, you were okay with the answer, but now you want more. You get what you can from the Web, and after a call to your doctor's office, you are inundated with information. As the office nurse robotically rattles off the details, you think to yourself, "Clearly, I'm not the only woman who isn't absorbing everything during the consultation."

Clomiphene citrate, or Clomid, is a pill taken to help you ovulate. That's great news for women who don't ovulate. But you're certain you ovulate every month; past blood tests have proven it. So why do you need a drug to help you ovulate? "It will help you ovulate better," is the response you get from the doctor. You immediately think, "How can a woman ovulate better?" Okay, now you feel like you're back in junior high school having an argument with your mother. The exchange goes something like this, "Just take it," your mother barks as she spoons an unknown green liquid into your mouth. "Why?" you spit back. "Because I said so, that's why," she replies as she spins on her heels and walks out of the room. The doctor may be more subtle, but the message is clearly the same.

If you already ovulate, Clomid may help you ovulate more eggs. Clomid triggers your brain to release FSH (follicle stimulating hormone) into your system. The ovary is stimulated by the FSH and begins producing estrogen, which helps a follicle grow. Your doctor will begin your Clomid treatment on day three, four or five of your cycle, and you will continue taking the drug for five days. Most doctors will suggest Clomid for three cycles, but in some cases it may be more.

I'll Have Clomid with a Side of Sweats

Your doctor warned you about the possible side effects of Clomid but said they might go unnoticed. Not much in the fertility world goes unnoticed, so you welcome the change. Irritability, mood swings, headaches and hot flashes are among the side effects, but you feel fairly moody these days anyway, and you're certainly not going to let a few night sweats deter you.

Another much less obvious side effect is the thinning of your uterine lining. Your doctor reassures you an ultrasound can be done to measure your lining and indicate if this is a problem. If it is, your doctor can prescribe medication that will help. Great! Another pill.

The consistency of your cervical fluid is once again called into question. Because Clomid causes it to thicken, you begin wondering to yourself, "When was the last time I thought so much about the consistency of anything? Hmmm, I guess that would be my ninth-grade Home Ec class and the day we learned how to make pancakes. Mrs. Holliday had really emphasized how important it was to get the batter just right. Too thin, it's like a crepe; too thick, you have a Belgian waffle. And so it is with your cervical fluid—if it's too thick, the sperm can't swim through to your cervix. If this is an issue, your doctor will most likely elect to do artificial insemination, a procedure that can bypass potential obstacles and boost your chances of pregnancy.

Artificial Insemination: It's as Real as It Gets

Remember when you first heard the words "artificial insemination"? We do too. These two words are not freely tossed around at barbecues and Sunday brunches, so you may be shocked and confused when you hear the words for the first time, especially if it sounds like it's going to be part of your treatment process. Just when you've gotten comfortable with the fact you are taking drugs to help you have a baby, you are faced with something that sounds really creepy. Before you can finish voicing your concern at the prospect of introducing something "artificial" to the whole process, your doctor dismisses the notion, telling you it's an extremely common procedure. Well, okay then. Moving right along.

We're convinced the medical world changed the terminology from artificial insemination to intrauterine insemination (IUI) to reduce the creep factor, making it seem more medical and less "artificial."

So what is an IUI exactly? When you reach the point of ovulation, your doctor will want to closely time your insemination. Essentially, you're giving sperm a free pass—sidestepping the cervix and directly escorting them into the uterus. Medically it all sounds great; emotionally you struggle. But after having a more thorough understanding, you realize it is not so much artificial; it's more a procedure to help give the sperm a boost and help them find their way a little more easily.

To maximize the IUI, a doctor will wash the sperm prior to the procedure to isolate the best sperm for the insemination. The sperm is placed in a centrifuge—essentially a high-tech salad spinner—to separate the good sperm from the not-so-good. The Olympic swimmers are left, and the doggie paddlers are tossed aside.

The IUI procedure is done in your doctor's office and feels much like a Pap smear. The vagina is opened with a speculum to visualize the cervix, and a small catheter containing the sperm is inserted through the cervical opening into the uterine cavity; the sperm are then deposited at the top of the uterus. During normal intercourse, a lot of sperm never make it past the cervix or get lost along the way. With an IUI, there is little room for error because the sperm are escorted to the right spot.

An IUI is kind of like kicking your golf ball out of the rough when nobody's looking. You want to get a clean shot, and in the end, nobody really needs to know anyway.

Some woman may experience mild cramping during and after the procedure, but it will not interfere with conception. Research varies on the success rates for IUI, but doctors agree that if you lack cervical fluid, if the fluid is too thick or if your husband has poor sperm quality, an IUI eliminates the problem.

And Away We Go

Finally, you give into the facts. You are not pregnant, and you don't want to continue trying on your own without help. You are ready to move into the world of fertility treatment, albeit the beginning stage. Somewhere buried inside those ovaries is a good egg, and you are bound and determined to find it! For the first time in quite a few months, you're excited about trying to get pregnant.

Fill'er Up, Please

You're officially starting fertility treatment! A claim you would have never dreamed of making in your attempts to bear children, but you have a rejuvenated attitude, and whatever it takes to get pregnant, you're willing to try. So it's off to the same apathetic, disinterested, grunge pharmacy where you purchase your monthly care package; you figure it's the best place to fill your Clomid prescription.

You deliver your doctor's slip to the drop-off window and quickly head to the Hallmark section to bury your face among the greeting cards. You thought it was embarrassing purchasing your monthly goods, but now you're in the big leagues, filling a fertility prescription. A few moments later, you see the pharmacist waving a piece of paper, clearly not using her "inside voice," saying, "Your insurance doesn't cover fertility drugs, okay?" Your mind is racing and a flash of anger spills over you; you're tempted to blurt out "Shut up, the entire store can hear you!" Instead, you hunch your shoulders, keep your head down and walk quickly back to the woman to inform her, "Yes, it's fine, whatever . . . just fill it." You find the nearest chair to collapse in, but after surveying the other occupants, you quickly realize the complimentary seating is reserved for the elderly and those with heart conditions. You jump to your feet, not wanting to draw any more unnecessary attention to yourself. Finally, your name is called, and you expect to see a few raised eyebrows as the pharmacist hands you the package. But much to your surprise, everyone gives you a soft smile. Pity? Sympathy? Possibly both. But as quickly as you sweep the pills off the counter and into your purse, you have erased it from your mind.

As you exit the pharmacy parking lot, you take a quick right turn and nearly run down a few local shoppers. Don't they understand? You are in a rush to get home and open your new prescription. You've never seen fertility drugs before, and your curiosity is piqued. When you open the brown plastic pill bottle, you are both disappointed and relieved to see there are only five tiny pills. For some reason, as you gaze into the vial, barely able to see the pills lost on the bottom, you feel like Alice in Wonderland looking down the rabbit hole. Oh well, hopefully the side effects will be as unimpressive as the pills.

Can so few pills really do so much? Maybe the pharmacist filled the wrong prescription and gave you Mrs. Applebaum's high blood pressure medication instead. Won't she be surprised when she ends up pregnant with twins next month? After carefully and thoroughly checking the label, you accept you have the correct medication. Well, no better time than the present—you swallow your first pill and wait for the effects.

Dr. Jekyll and Mrs. Hyde

Some of our TTCs claim they had little or no side effects while on Clomid. They took the pills and didn't notice erratic moods or hot flashes. We hope you fall into this category and avoid any notable physical reaction. Other TTCs claim petulance much like a cornered rat. Of the most commonly reported side effects, mood swings and irritability top the charts. Be warned: the side effects tend to creep up on you. If you start looking for signs on the first day, you won't find any. However, on day three or four, you may begin to notice some bad behavior, for instance, yelling obscenities at the woman who stole your parking space at the supermarket or having a screaming match with your toddler over the green crayon she used to scribble on your freshly painted wall. Your husband may also notice a change in your disposition, but if he is smart, he will keep his mouth shut and his wallet open. A note to husbands: avoid all confrontational subjects and order take-out often. Even better, make a reservation, and take your wife out to dinner.

If you find yourself watching sappy preteen TV with tear-filled eyes, you are probably a little more sensitive than usual. This enhanced emotional you is courtesy of Clomid. It could be your neighbor's graduation, a friend's wedding or even two strangers on the street embraced in a kiss; it won't take much to make you weepy. You can safely assume all unexplained reactions are a result of Clomid.

As you take great efforts to keep your emotions intact, you analyze your situation. Would my reaction be the same if I were taking a placebo? Am I really this sad, hopeless and angry about my situation, or is it the Clomid talking? Am I extra crazy this month because the side effects of Clomid say I will be? As soon as your mood shifts to a happier place or you wake up in the night drenched in sweat, you realize no, this is not a placebo, and yes, you are experiencing huge hormonal swings and surges. As frustrating as the side effects may be, your unrelenting desire to have a baby is still your top priority. You can live with a few outbursts, and the hot flashes are just a sneak preview of what lies ahead with menopause. However, if your emotions get the best of you, and your irritability is beyond control, you should consult your doctor.

Take Five Clomid and Call Me When You Ovulate

You're down to the last pill on the fifth and final day. Whew, at least that part is over. The next few days will be spent tracking your ovulation. Depending on your doctor, this will be done one of two ways. Some doctors will have you use ovulation predictor sticks to start testing for your LH surge around day seven. Yes, those sticks are back to plague you once again. When the stick goes off, you will return to your doctor's office the next morning for an IUI.

Alternately, a more hands-on doctor will forego the ovulation sticks; a few days after you finish Clomid, he will have you come to the office for a vaginal ultrasound. This is an ultrasound you will welcome with open legs because you will be anxious to see the results. With all of the emotional ups and downs you've endured, you figure you should have at least a dozen eggs ready to go. The ultrasound will show how many follicles are growing; each follicle should carry an egg. The more eggs you release in a given month, the better your chances of becoming pregnant that month. Depending on your reaction to the medication, your doctor will want to see one mature follicle or, in some cases, two or more. Based on the size of your follicles, the doctor will have a good indication of when you will ovulate.

Regardless of the tracking method, and to leave nothing to

chance, once the follicles are mature, your doctor may give you an injection of human chorionic gonadotropin (hCG). This injection is given to stimulate ovulation, which should occur between twelve and thirty-six hours later. If you receive the shot in the morning, you will return to the office for an IUI the next day.

Give Me Everything You've Got

On the day of your vaginal ultrasound, you leave the doctor's office with a small brown bag that contains a sterile plastic cup. Wrapped around the cup are very specific instructions for the semen collection. The morning of the semen collection, while pouring the coffee and with a smirk plastered on your face, you hand the bag over to your husband. You smile because you have read the instructions and know, more or less, you are off the hook. Your husband is about to find out sperm collection is a very private matter. He may have been in a better mood today if his attempts at having sex last night had been reciprocated. During the 11:00 news commercial break, however, his playful advances were mercilessly denied. You shot him down, not because you didn't want to have a late-night romp but because your doctor gave you specific instructions NOT to have sex the day before your IUI. Handing him the cup and the instructions for semen collection seals the deal. He is officially irritated. He looks to you for help as he sees your eyes scroll down the list to instruction #4:

> It is preferred that the semen specimen be collected by masturbation in a private room located in our office. Masturbation is preferable to coitus interruptus (interrupted sexual intercourse) because the latter may result in loss of the first portion of ejaculate. A semen collection kit is available if intercourse is needed.

He's on his own with this one. You do, however, feel a twinge of sympathy and point out instruction #7:

> If the specimen cannot be collected in our office, it should be collected in the proper container noting the date and time of collection and the last date of intercourse. The specimen must be protected from cold or heat during transport to the laboratory (place the semen container in a shirt pocket or area next to the body for proper warmth). The specimen must be delivered to the laboratory within forty-five minutes after collection. If it cannot, then it must be collected in our office.

The last sentence gives your husband the nudge he needs to head back to the bathroom to perform his duties. You feel a twinge of empathy and then remind yourself that your vagina will soon be the hot spot hosting doctors, nurses and sperm. When your husband returns to the kitchen with his plastic cup in hand, he mumbles something like, "This just isn't good timing for me." You ignore the comment and try to keep a straight face as he declares, "It's kind of a small amount. I must be tired." You decide not to bruise his male ego and break the news that he is normal and that the amount (about the size of a teaspoon) is a standard ejaculation.

One TTC actually said her husband gives new meaning to "his cup runneth over," claiming his container was overflowing when he provided his sperm sample. We're pretty certain this is a fabrication of his virility, but give her major kudos for building up her "man's manhood."

It takes, on average, about seventy-two hours for sperm to develop, and because your husband is always making new sperm, his semen may not always be consistent, so sample sizes may vary slightly. You could tell your husband all of this, but it would fall on deaf ears—his part of the relay is done. He is out the door, not giving it a second thought.

Ready, Aim, Fire

"Thanks," you reply as you're handed the same paper gown you receive at every visit. You confirm with the nurse—yes, the sperm she is holding on a sterile tray is your husband's. Suddenly, you flash back to another appointment. You are sitting in the waiting area, and several nurses are whispering as they surround the "Welcome to the World" photo montage filled with newborn pictures, birth announcements and Christmas cards. Obviously intended to be a visual inspiration to their newer patients, the wall promises hope to women who enter the clinic doors empty-handed that they may one day leave with a baby in their arms. A beautiful image? Yes. But what haunts you is the nurse's conversation you recall overhearing. "The Martin twins look nothing like the mother." "Or father," another chimes in. Your stomach drops. Oh my God—did they mix up the semen sample?

Sitting in your paper nightie, you are filled with fear that the nurse has somehow mistakenly switched your husband's semen sample with the McGillacuddy's, and you will be giving birth to a set of flaming redheads. You shake the vision from your mind. When you mention your concerns to the nurse, she assures you there are multiple checkpoints in place to ensure this would never happen.

Your doctor enters the room, explains the procedure and, without haste, begins his work: "You'll feel a slight pinch, but try to relax." You ask yourself, "How am I supposed to relax with you perched in my crotch shooting my husband's sperm into my uterus?" Your eyes tear up, and you think to yourself, I should be at home in our bedroom making love with my husband, making a baby the good old-fashioned way, not in a sterile room with two people I barely know.

You force yourself to think positively. Even though your

husband is not sharing the physical experience with you, his words help. Prior to the IUI, you called to share your anxiety, and he gave you his best pep talk. "Try to think good thoughts," he said. "I'm pretty sure we covered our bases and you're already pregnant. Think of the insemination as a safety net." Sweet, and he's right too. Since sperm can live for days in cervical fluid, his little guys have been hanging around waiting for your egg to fall. Maybe he has been listening. You end the conversation with, "Thanks. I love you, and I'll call you later."

Cigarette?

Much more quickly than you thought, the whole thing is over. Your husband's swift at times, but never this speedy. The nurse reaches for the egg timer on the counter, turns the dial to ten and says, "You've got ten minutes to relax. When the timer goes off, get dressed, and you're free to go home." Great—the fertility version of *Beat the Clock.* You drop your head to the pillow and force yourself to relax, again.

Comforted that the IUI is over, you are able to settle your thoughts. If only they offered a foot rub and shoulder massage, this wouldn't be so bad. You try to envision the sperm swimming wildly toward your egg and one of them beating the door down. You could be pregnant this very moment! Okay, minus the pinching, this could possibly be the best baby sex you've had.

In reality, the past months have been tense, and ovulation has always put an extra strain on your bedroom activities. This wasn't so bad, but your heart pangs a little when you think about the romantic alternative: at home, cuddled in your husband's arms, surrounded by candles instead of lying motionless on a cold hard table with your feet suspended in stirrups. The timer dings, and you snap back to reality. You get dressed and make a beeline for the door. You're a little uncomfortable at what's just happened but relieved it's finally over.

Is That All There Is?

After the appointment, you find yourself standing in line at the FedEx office looking around and wondering, "Do these people know I just had an IUI?" Unbelievably, just hours before, you were experiencing what you considered to be an enormous moment in your life. Fast forward. You are out and about, running mundane errands. How can something that was so monumental in the weeks leading up to it now seem anticlimactic?

You wonder if there is any way you could have made the "event" more special or magical? You wish you had brought your husband along, but since there wasn't much he could do, you thought you'd go it alone this time. But now you're thinking, if you do end up pregnant, it would have been great to at least have him in the room when it happened.

Over the next week, you find you are less preoccupied with getting pregnant and feel more positive about being pregnant. A welcome change that leaves you inspired instead of stressed. You spend a great deal of time reflecting on your doctor's comments that this was an excellent cycle, perfect in fact. When you asked about the next steps, he almost inferred this could be the month. You can't wait to find out, but for now you are happy to be pill-free.

To: Patty <Patty@conceptionchronicles.com>;
           Shelly <Shelly@conceptionchronicles.com>
From: Courtney <Courtney@conceptionchronicles.com>
Subject: **Ski trip**

Are you guys both in for the ski trip? We need to finalize the reservation for the house.

To: Courtney <Courtney@conceptionchronicles.com>;
           Shelly <Shelly@conceptionchronicles.com>
From: Patty <Patty@conceptionchronicles.com>
Subject: **RE: Ski Trip**

Sorry it's taken me so long to get back to you. I've been dragging my feet b/c I may have to start injectible drugs if Clomid doesn't work. It's a much more demanding process.

Scott and I talked about it last night, and he said we can't let fertility treatments rule our lives . . . so we're coming! Count us in! If it does come down to that, I'll ask my <u>NEW</u> doctor (whom I love) if I can have my blood taken in Vail and fax the results back to his office. I'm sure it will all work out.

To: Courtney <Courtney@conceptionchronicles.com>;
           Patty <Patty@conceptionchronicles.com>
From: Shelly <Shelly@conceptionchronicles.com>
Subject: **RE: RE: Ski Trip**

Count us in too. I can't wait to see you guys! See you on the slopes!

chapter nine

The Envelope, Please

Wednesday   Notes

- Buy pregnancy tests

Thursday   Notes   **Friday**   Notes

- Drugstore
- Tissues
- Candy
- Ovulation sticks

- Rent Terms of Endearment

- Find a therapist

Ask any woman trying to get pregnant where she is in her current cycle, and she will rattle off the exact day (day nine), her ovulation date (Tuesday the twenty-third) and the number of days until her next expected period (nineteen, not including today). These stats are burned in her brain much like the typical male who has every batting average of his favorite baseball team readily available for a spontaneous game of sports trivia.

For those of us who live for colored filing systems and home-office label makers, the ovulation cycle can be neatly compartmentalized into two-week units. The two weeks leading up to ovulation involve frantic monitoring, serious sexual activity and huge hormonal swings; super-size the hormonal swings if you have started taking fertility drugs. The two weeks following ovulation include serious nail biting and hyperanalyzing every sign and symptom of a potential pregnancy. The two-week wait (known notoriously as "2ww" on the bulletin boards) leading up to your period is an excruciating, emotional chapter in the odyssey of having a child. As the months pass by and your efforts to get pregnant become more aggressive, the 2ww becomes more punishing with each fruitless effort.

It's incredible how much your emotions may sink and soar during the 2ww. It's important to note these manic tendencies are not reserved for those taking fertility drugs. Any woman trying to have a baby for an extended period of time will likely exhibit obsessive behavior during the 2ww. One day you are overwhelmed with happiness, absolutely convinced you are pregnant. Twenty-four hours later, your mood swerves dramatically, and you are drowning in disappointment and despair that another month will pass you by without a pregnancy. Fourteen days can feel like fourteen months as your emotions ebb and flow like the Atlantic tides before a spring hurricane hits shore.

Fourteen Days and Counting

Every woman's emotional roller coaster will have its own personal peaks and valleys mixed in with a variety of twists, turns and "loop to loops." Much like a tumultuous ride on a monstrous coaster, it's sometimes hard to tell if you are up or down during the 2ww. Here's a quick day-by-day snapshot of a typical internal dialogue during the 2ww:

DPO = (Day Post Ovulation)

1 DPO: This is going to be the month. I know it.

2 DPO: We should have sex one more time tonight, just to be sure.

3 DPO: I don't want to ruin this perfect cycle. We'll have sex again this morning, just in case.

4 DPO: We did it. Everything was perfect.

5 DPO: Whew . . . it's over. We did everything we possibly could do.

6 DPO: I wish we hadn't skipped sex on day ten, but sperm can live for a couple of days, right?

7 DPO: Forget it; who am I kidding? I'm not pregnant. I can see a big pimple in the middle of my forehead. I'm having a glass of wine.

8 DPO: I'm never going to be a mother.

9 DPO: Wait, I feel different. Maybe I will be a mother.

10 DPO: My boobs are really sore, and I'm so tired.

11 DPO: I'm definitely pregnant!

12 DPO: What was I thinking drinking that wine? My baby's going to have brain damage.

13 DPO: No sign of my period. That's it . . . I'm pregnant. I'm taking a test tomorrow.

14 DPO: Negative. But it's still really early to get an accurate response. My back aches—I wonder what that means?

15 DPO: Spotting. It doesn't mean anything. I'm taking another test. Hmmm, this one looks different. Where's my flashlight? I need to get a better look.

16 DPO: Another test; another negative. Crap. But I still don't have my period, so there's still hope. Why did I cheap out and buy these generic tests? I'll try a different brand tomorrow.

CD = (Cycle Day)

CD1: Oh, God! How can this be happening again? I got my period.

CD2: Forget the pinot grigio. I need a cosmo.

Where Ovulation Ends, Speculation Begins

Each month, you manage to convince yourself this will be "the month." You believe this with all your heart because there really isn't a good reason why you shouldn't get pregnant. You tracked your ovulation meticulously, religiously popped your Clomid, engaged in bona fide sex with your husband precisely when you needed to and even when you didn't, and you went the extra yard with another round of IUI. Everything was perfect. Even your reproductive endocrinologist who supervised your every move agreed—it all looked great. This will be the month.

You think back to when two weeks in your life seemed to just fly by—the last days of summer vacation, the first weeks getting to know a new boyfriend, the date your library book is due. Why are these fourteen days so unbearable? Why do they pass more slowly than a kidney stone working its way through your bladder?

Is It Real or Is It Memorex?

Once ovulation is confirmed, the countdown begins. And to add to your already borderline insanity, your mind now begins to play tricks on your body. You know the pregnancy symptoms you want to experience—sore boobs, fatigue, an acute sense of smell. You chronically look for all of them. Walks in the produce aisle not only include fondling the fruit for freshness but also a sly grope of your own breast in search of tenderness. You pass time at traffic lights pressing and grabbing each boob, very much to the liking of the old man in the car next to you. Your morning shower includes a daily souped-up breast exam, and you even sneak in a poke here and there at work while staring at your computer. Yes, your breasts ache this month, but why? Because you're pregnant? Because you're getting your period? Or is it because you've been poking at them for the past five days?

You've always been hypersensitive to odors. You could detect the stench of spoiled milk with the refrigerator door closed. Now you convince yourself your sense of smell has intensified further, and you can sniff out the most innocuous scents. This is definitely a good sign, since you clearly remember your sister-in-law could not stand to be around even the mildest perfumes when she was pregnant.

Cyber Support

While you will always rely on your inner circle of friends for support and information, many of them may not be able to help you because they just don't have all the answers. Even those who have been through the fertility wringer seem to block out the mundane details of the process once they achieve success. Just like mothers can't recall the pain of childbirth, many women labeled "infertile" can't remember the pain they had to endure before reaching their dreams.

When urgent questions pop to mind in the middle of the night during your 2ww, there's always a place you can turn. The fertility bulletin boards—open nights, weekends and holidays. There are many out there, and with a little effort, you'll discover you're not alone. There is a whole community of women in the same situation. Many of the chat rooms are organized by age, diagnosis and treatment. So if you're a twenty-five-year-old woman with blocked fallopian tubes and are about to have your first IUI, there will be thirty other women exactly like you just a click away, waiting to offer their support.

You'll probably notice a definite shift in your interest in the fertility-related Web sites. In the past, you were searching for facts and figures, and good old reliable Google did the trick. Now you're not so concerned about the general population; you're concerned about you. Do other women have spotting before they get their period like you do? Do tender breasts really mean this could be the month? This is crucial information you must know—today! While the bulletin boards are great for answering the questions you already have, be warned that they will also open the floodgates to millions of questions you never knew to ask. Your posted question about premenstrual spotting opens up a whole new discussion around "implantation spotting." This is news to you, but apparently when the embryo is implanting in the uterus, a woman can experience spotting. Your new cyber friends tell you to hold on to your hope this month. The spotting you are experiencing may very well be a sign of your little guy settling in and getting comfortable for his nine-month nap.

It's Better to Be Safe Than Sorry

The immediate days following your ovulation find you in a fertile frenzy. Although your doctor has confirmed you have done everything you could this month to optimize your chances of pregnancy, you are not entirely certain. When you ask your doctor for one more ultrasound just to confirm the follicles released the eggs, he flatly denies you. "The hCG trigger shot leaves nothing to chance," he says. You know your ovulation was perfectly coordinated with an IUI, but you want to cover all your bases, so you will maintain your Code Red sex schedule for the next few days. Who knows? Maybe the egg popped out a bit late, and you don't want to take any chances of screwing up this cycle.

Still not willing to let it go, you think to yourself, "What harm can a little extra sex do?" Unfortunately and unbelievably, your husband does not concur. Between all of his sex-on-demand performances and the high-pressure homework assignment he had for the IUI, he's had enough. As usual, you are relentless, and he reluctantly concedes. He simply can't risk the odds of your being right—even if those odds are less than his chances of marrying a supermodel in his next life.

Play, Stop, Rewind

By day four post ovulation (4DPO), you've resigned yourself to the fact that, this month, your fate in becoming a mother no longer rests in your hands but with a higher power. You're relieved and liberated. It's over. There is nothing more you can do. And while you've accepted you cannot do a thing to impact this month's tremendous efforts, you can't stop recapping, replaying and redoing every sexual encounter you had before, during and after ovulation.

You've booted your husband from his leather La-Z-Boy and comfortably settled in to spend the next few days reviewing the game tapes and criticizing this month's Operation Ovulation play-book. Maybe you should have had sex every other day instead of every day. You wonder if that last-minute business trip of yours screwed up your schedule. You hope the sperm were strong enough, even though your doctor reassured you the sample was above average.

Amazingly, your husband is happy to give up his recliner. No wonder—he instead propositions you to meet him in the bedroom. Apparently, his oversexed self has regained his libido, and he's ready for some postgame action. You, on the other hand, could be no less interested. At this point, you feel like you've had enough sex in the past few weeks to last you a lifetime. For now, you are happy to sit on the sidelines.

Fertility Folklore

Sex during the 2ww is a hot topic among your cyberfriends on the bulletin boards. While the orgasm is credited with helping to "pull" the sperm into the uterus during ovulation, the big "O" has a much different rap sheet after ovulation. Some claim that an orgasm dur-ing the 2ww can actually prevent pregnancy. When you hear the argu-ment that the contractions during an orgasm may cause an embryo to dislodge from the uterus if it is not firmly implanted, you actu-ally think it makes sense. The thought conjures up California living, where bookshelves and china cabinets are anchored to the wall to protect the precious contents from unexpected tremors.

We grew up reading *Cosmopolitan* magazine and were taught the whole point of having sex was to have an orgasm (multiple if you're very industrious and have a little extra time on your hands). Over the years, some of your girlfriends had confessed they rarely, if ever, achieved orgasm. You always felt sorry for them and never thought you'd be envious of their unconscious libido, until now. As you think back to those conversations and realize today they are all driving monstrous SUVs, complete with a third-row seat to accommodate their ever-expanding families, you think there really may be something to the "O" theory.

You set your embarrassment aside and decide to ask your doctor. At the end of your next appointment, you start fidgeting while working up the courage to discuss the dangers of good sex during the 2ww. After a few moments of awkward silence, your doctor asks, "Is there anything else?" There's no time like the present. You just spit it out, "Could an orgasm be preventing me from getting pregnant?"

"Where did you hear something as ridiculous as that?" he replies with the look of someone who thought he heard everything until you pulled this pearl of wisdom out of your hat. When you tell him it's the latest information flying around cyberspace, he replies, "There's some crazy stuff on the Internet." Of course, you value the opinion of a man who spent eight years in medical school and countless years in practice, but you still can't shake the feeling there may be something to this.

When your husband gets home, you can't wait to share the ultimate irony—your good sex life may be preventing you from getting pregnant. This is just too much for him. He was a good sport when you removed caffeine, alcohol, chocolate and soybeans from your life, but now you're saying you no longer want to enjoy physical contact during the two weeks when sex actually has no other purpose than pleasure and offers a chance to reconnect after the torture of sex on demand.

You tell him you're not going that far—of course you can still have intercourse; you just need to take it down a notch. Under no circumstance is he to perform his secret weapon move that gets you every time. Even though it's taken years for him to perfect, and he's more than impressed with its guaranteed results, for now it's off the menu—at least until you ovulate again and need the extra boost to get his sperm where they need to go.

To: Shelly <Shelly@conceptionchronicles.com>
From: Patty <Patty@conceptionchronicles.com>
Cc: Courtney <Courtney@conceptionchronicles.com>
Subject: **Two words . . .**

Eat pineapple.

To: Patty <Patty@conceptionchronicles.com>
From: Shelly <Shelly@conceptionchronicles.com>
Cc: Courtney <Courtney@conceptionchronicles.com>
Subject: **Re: Two words . . .**

I know.

I read the same thing on the bulletin board. I'm not sure how it could possibly help me get pregnant, but who cares. I'm on my third one in two days. I have a sore on my tongue the size of a quarter from all the acid, but I'm chewing around it and not giving up.

To: Patty <Patty@conceptionchronicles.com>;
           Shelly <Shelly@conceptionchronicles.com>
From: Courtney <Courtney@conceptionchronicles.com>
Subject: **Re: Re: Two words . . .**

Good God.

I'm sure it's hard not to jump on every BB bandwagon, but keep in mind, moderation is key. I guess it can't hurt, but don't make yourselves crazy. Next week's fertility food favorite might be something far less appealing, like boiled cabbage.

Are We There Yet?

Midway through the 2ww, your postgame analysis has you apt to believe that this will not be the month your life will be changed forever. Despite the progesterone test you took to confirm you did indeed ovulate, you are certain you are not pregnant. Maybe it's a natural defense mechanism, but it's the only way you know how to manage your soaring expectations. You slip back into your normal, nonovulating, not-pregnant life. You splurge and have your latte fully loaded when your favorite coffee spot is out of decaf; you go crazy and have a couple glasses of pinot grigio at book club; you even stop overdosing on pineapple or the fertility food du jour.

You Gotta Be in It to Win It

As easily as you were able to convince yourself you could not possibly be pregnant, the next moment your convictions make a 180-degree turn, and you allow yourself to dream again. Maybe, just maybe, you are. Your breasts hurt, but not in the same way they do when you're getting your period. Was that a gas pain you just felt? No, it must have been the embryo implanting in your uterus. Women feel that happening, right? You log on to the bulletin board and are happy to see other women reporting the same "symptoms."

Well then, that's it. You are definitely pregnant. You can see yourself sporting a cute little belly just in time for the holidays. Of course you're pregnant; you did everything right this month. Your doctor verified you ovulated, and he personally escorted your husband's handpicked sperm to the right place, at the right time. You dash to the drug store and purchase a five-day advance pregnancy test. However, at home, in the privacy of your bathroom, you debate taking it. At the same moment, you're both excited and terrified to confirm or deny your chances of motherhood.

Where Speculation Ends, Rationalization Begins

Your solitary heart-to-heart goes something like this, "If the test is positive, I promise with all of my heart I will be the best mother any child could ever hope to have. But if it's negative, it's not the end of the world. I could still be pregnant; it's still a little early to be testing." You rip the wrapper open.

There are only two days until your expected period, and there is still no sign of its arrival. Eighty percent of your free time is spent on the toilet. You are keeping Carefree Panty Shields in business. You are scrutinizing every drop of fluid on your panty liner, examining it closely for even the slightest tinge of bright red. If you had a microscope handy, you'd use it. Things are really looking good. Then it hits you. Your recent "unmotherly" behavior comes back to haunt you. You should never have had that extra glass of wine. What were you thinking? What if your baby has brain damage? You're already a terrible mother.

You Ain't Seen Nothing Yet

Fourteen days since ovulation, and still no sign of your "friend." It's back to the drugstore; this time for a bulk supply of pregnancy tests. And you thought you could blow through ovulation sticks— that was child's play compared with the obsessive testing you carry on now. One of our TTCs actually bought four different brands of pregnancy tests. When she got home, she lined them up on the bathroom counter and, one by one, took each test until she exhausted her supply. She was looking for inconsistencies in the test, but even more than that, she was looking for just one of these tests to deliver the result she so desperately wanted. Who cares if three tests tell you you're not pregnant—if one comes back positive, the others are clearly wrong.

Each time the results are negative, you tell yourself it must be too early to tell. You want so badly to be pregnant, and with no apparent sign you're not, you actually tell your husband things are looking good. He is so excited, he bends down to talk to your tummy and welcomes "your little one" to the family. Your heart silently breaks.

A few days pass and the familiar premenstrual symptoms start to appear, but you choose to ignore them. Your face breaks out; it must be your new skin cream. The cramps kick in; it must be something you ate. You're bloated; pregnant women get bloated too. To spare your husband from another disappointment, you start to slowly break the news as each telltale sign appears that you don't think this is the month. When you tell him you think you're going to get your period at any minute, he does his best to cheer you on and tells you, "It ain't over 'til it's over."

In spite of what you tell your husband and all of the routine indications, you consider yourself period-free until the full flow arrives in all of its Technicolor glory. Any spotting, regardless of the hue, is attributed to your extra-sluggish embryo taking its sweet time to implant itself in your uterus. You sustain fanatical testing, which yields the same results over and over and over again—negative. Reality is banging on the bathroom door, but you hold on to any glimmer of hope you have left. Until the moment the crimson tide actually arrives, you honestly believe there is a chance you are pregnant.

The Worst Day of My Life: Take Two, Three, Four, Five . . .

Then it happens. Your worst nightmare comes true—you get your period . . . again. You crumble to your knees and, on the cold marble floor, burst into tears, your body sobbing. How could this happen? You did everything right. You were under medical supervision and were told by a trained professional your cycle was perfect. What could have gone wrong? Your head is spinning, but the only explanation you can even remotely conjure up was the morning sex session you skipped on day ten. Incredible, one tiny mistake, and this is what happens. If you didn't get pregnant this month, it must mean you never will. You feel completely alone, hopeless, desperate. The thought of breaking the news to your husband makes you want to throw up.

You can't take it anymore. How can you possibly go through this again next month? This was your third attempt to get pregnant on Clomid, and as you know, three strikes and you're out. You are exhausted and swear off taking any more drugs that make you act like a lunatic. The thought of having mandatory sex for ten straight days literally makes your skin crawl. Maybe you just weren't meant to be a mother. It shouldn't be this hard. In the background, you hear the phone ringing, but you can't imagine having a conversation without crying, especially since it's probably just a telemarketer peddling low-interest-rate mortgages. You feel like your life is over.

To: Courtney <Courtney@conceptionchronicles.com>;
         Shelly <Shelly@conceptionchronicles.com>
From: Patty <Patty@conceptionchronicles.com>
Subject: **This sucks!**

I'm so depressed. I just got my period. Not only do I have to start shooting up next month with fertility drugs, but I called my doctor to run by my "remote ski vacation" treatment plan, and he said absolutely not. Apparently there's more to this process than slipping off the slopes for a quick blood test.

I can't believe it's come to this. My entire life is ruled by our attempts to have a baby. This will be the second time our money is going on vacation without us!

To:	Patty <Patty@conceptionchronicles.com>
From:	Courtney <Courtney@conceptionchronicles.com>
Cc:	Shelly <Shelly@conceptionchronicles.com>
Subject:	**RE: This sucks!**

What a bummer!!! I told Dan the bad news, and if you can believe it, he asked if Scott could still come alone. I said, "Sure, if Scott wants to spend the rest of his life <u>alone</u>." It won't be the same w/out you, but we'll raise a hot toddy in your honor.

If I Could Read Minds, I'd Be a Millionaire

Your husband's reaction to your recurring bad news is never quite what you want it to be. Poor guy; he simply does not know what to do or say. Even after months of disappointment, he can never seem to get it right. Men and women typically express themselves very differently when the emotional stakes are high. Men tend to be much less emotional and much more rational, which is why they live on Mars and we live on Venus. And to be fair, if you've spent the last few days telling your husband you don't think you are pregnant while you secretly hoped and prayed you were, he is responding to the only information you've given him. When you call him at the office and tell him through a cracked voice that you've gotten your period, he may calmly reply you knew it was coming and then try to comfort you by saying you can always try again next month. As you listen to him, you know he's right, but you just can't understand why he isn't as upset as you are. Doesn't he want this as much as you do?

It's sometimes hard to remember, but he's enduring his own version of the emotional roller coaster you ride together each month. You are perched in the front seat, preparing yourself for each breathtaking climb and each stomach-dropping descent as you see them approaching. He is trailing far behind in the last car dragged by your momentum, oblivious to each rise and fall until they've already begun.

His entire body may not be experiencing what your body is, but his heart and soul are equally invested in having a baby. Still, you can't understand why he is not completely simpatico with you . . . mood for mood, hope for hope, tear for tear. Remember, he does not spend the 2ww overanalyzing his body for every cramp, pain and phantom symptom of pregnancy. So give the fella a break, and instead try to understand that he is doing the best he can to keep it together for you and for him.

Also remember that he's not the only support you have. It's a good time to turn to your good old reliable girlfriends. Whether they've been through the process personally or not, they always manage to find the perfect combination of support and sympathy you need.

I'll Take Conception for $500, Alex

The day you get your period is now so emotionally and physically draining you've unconsciously created a survival routine just to get through it. After digging out the super-size tampons from your bathroom cabinet, you finally admit defeat. You are not pregnant. So you do what you've done every month on this god-awful day. It's barely noon, but you call it quits. A mental health day, and you deserve it. You close the bedroom door, flip on the TV and settle into your big, comfy bed where you'll spend the next twelve hours watching reruns of *Jeopardy* on the Game Show Network. You happen to be quite the *Jeopardy* junkie, and correctly answering challenging, albeit inane, trivia questions for several hours is just what you need to feel useful and worthwhile. You may not be pregnant, but damn it, you're smart.

Is There a Doctor in the House?

It's perfectly normal to feel depressed when you get your period and realize another cycle has failed. Before you can gear yourself up for the next month's activities, you must mourn the loss of what could have been. Go ahead and throw yourself a big pity party, complete with a new pair of shoes, your favorite dessert and a movie rental that's guaranteed to get the tears flowing.

However, sometimes it's easy to start the tears but hard to stop them. Bearing the emotional burden of infertility can become completely overwhelming, whether or not you have a support system. If you start to realize you're feeling out of control, don't be embarrassed to seek the help you need.

Your doctor will likely be able to recommend a therapist who specializes in fertility issues. While the therapist will not be able to change the outcome of each month's efforts, she will be able to help you make the process more manageable. Simply having someone tell you what you're feeling is normal is a huge relief.

A therapist can also help you and your husband work through the issues as a couple. The only way to make it through the fertility minefields with your marriage intact is with constant communication. Although it sounds basic, sometimes a neutral third party is the catalyst you need to spark a discussion around the topics you may choose to ignore on your own.

Whether you choose to seek counseling individually or with your husband, you'll be glad you took the step and got the help you needed.

If at First You Don't Succeed, Try, Try Again

After you pick yourself up and get back on track, you realize you have but a day or two before the madness begins all over again. How are you ever going to do it? Well, this ain't your first rodeo, and you are able to shake off your sadness and despair and get back on the horse again. You are certainly not giving up your chances of becoming a mother, and the only thing you know how to do is move forward. All of the negative energy is now redirected toward hope and optimism. It's back to the playbook for this month's version of the Ovulation Olympics. Certainly, if trying to get pregnant were a sport, you'd be considered a world-class competitor—professionally trained and perfectly conditioned to succeed even under the most demanding circumstances.

It certainly has been a long road up until this point, but you've survived. You have no idea what's in store for you from here, but you know one way or another, you'll make it through.

chapter ten

Give It Your Best Shot

Saturday   Notes

- 11 a.m. injection class

Sunday   Notes   **Monday**   Notes

- Check price of
twin crib set @
Pottery Barn
Kids

After three months of mental meltdowns, you are more than happy to abandon Clomid and graduate to the next level of treatment. As you do every month, you set up an appointment with your doctor to review the previous cycle and discuss your options for the upcoming month. Of course, you always hope for some insight as to why things didn't work out, but you never seem to get it. Rather, you hear the same thing month after month from your doctor, "It was a good cycle. I was very happy with it." How could he possibly be happy with a cycle that didn't end with your sending out birth announcements? You couldn't care less if everything "looked" great; something clearly wasn't right, and you want to know what it is.

When you push your doctor for an explanation, you expect a reassuring speech about how it may be just a matter of time, and there's no need to worry. Instead, he tells you that until you do IVF and they can actually see the sperm interact with the egg, they may not be able to make an official diagnosis. The doctor starts listing things that potentially could be wrong, but the one that's burnt permanently in your memory is "bad egg quality." Don't panic when your doctor nonchalantly tosses out the notion you may never have a biological child. Almost every one of our TTCs going through the process has heard the same thing, regardless of whether her blood work indicated a problem.

If you have a solid diagnosis, like a low sperm count or an elevated FSH, you may not consider yourself lucky, but at least the treatment options will be tailored to your condition. For infertility patients who fall into the "unexplained" category, the process of treatment is not always so clear. Your doctor will make recommendations, but for the most part, the decision on how to proceed will be left up to you.

Local or Express?

"You have a choice to make," the doctor says, as he flings open a drawer and whips out a photocopied sheet of paper with a one-dimensional image of your reproductive parts. He starts spelling out the differences between using follicle stimulating hormones (FSH) with IUI (choice number one) and using in vitro fertilization (choice number two), all while referring back to your black-and-white uterus like an electronic chalkboard. Arrows, Xs and Os detail the plan to pull off the quarterback sneak and ultimately unite egg and sperm.

Both sound scary, but since you've already been through an IUI, you decide to take the less-aggressive step and try the follicle stimulating drugs before moving on to IVF. The success rates are significantly higher with IVF, but so is the cost, and quite frankly, you've always thought of IVF as a last resort. At this point, you don't even know if you would consider such an aggressive procedure. Hopefully, these drugs will do the trick, and you won't ever have to face that decision.

Once you announce your decision, the doctor starts rattling off information about the drugs, and you understand, on average, every third word out of his mouth. But in typical fashion, you do the uh-huh nod throughout his five-minute dissertation. Reality doesn't set in until he says, "There's a class you'll have to take to learn how to give yourself injections." INJECTIONS?! How could this have slipped your mind? You're sure he mentioned it in your initial consultation, but like a trauma victim, you completely suppressed any memory involving shots being given by anyone other than a trained medical professional.

You know there are millions of people around the world who give themselves injections (some recreationally), but you never thought you'd be one of them. You steered clear of the most innocent drugs in college primarily because you feared they would instantly catapult you into addict status, and the next thing you know, you'd be using your panty hose as a tourniquet and shooting up behind Taco Bell. But now, here you are, drug-free with a record clean enough to run for president, and you're about to learn how to "take a hit." It just doesn't seem fair.

When you finally work up the courage to call and set up an appointment for the injection class, the nurse tells you she can squeeze you into a group next week, but it may be longer if your husband wants to join you. If faced with this situation, there's only one thing to do—WAIT! Even if it takes three weeks, your husband really needs to be with you for this one, especially if he's going to be the one giving the shots. Up until this point, you've been completely considerate of his schedule and tried to tough it through as many tests and treatments on your own. Now's the time to lay down the law. There are no excuses. Even if the class is in the middle of the day, three hours away from his office, he needs to be there.

The New Drop/Add: I'd Like to Drop Pilates and Add FSH Injections

Regardless of how long you've waited, the day of your class arrives with shocking speed. As you walk into the waiting area of the doctor's office, it's painfully clear who is there for the injection class and who is there for a routine visit. The injection class students stand out like freshman on the first day of high school as they nervously clutch the information packet the receptionist hands them when they check in at the front desk. The other patients in the room are evenly split between those early in the process, the hand-holding couples who stare dreamily at the baby photo wall while whispering and giggling together and the slightly more sea-soned couples.

One of the latter, "been around the fertility block" couples looks a bit more weathered, at least the woman does. When the receptionist calls their name and the husband remains firmly seated in his chair long enough to finish the article he is reading in *Sports Illustrated*, his wife shoots him a glaring look that is all too familiar.

You never thought you'd have waiting room envy or that you would long for the early days of your treatment, but oh, how you do. You look at the nonclass patients and wonder what's in store for them this afternoon? Blood work? Vaginal ultrasound? IUI? You'd take it. Hands down. Anything other than sitting in a class learn-ing how to INJECT yourself with a NEEDLE!

The size of your doctor's medical practice will have a tremen-dous influence on your actual class experience. If you're with one of those "best in the country" practices in New York City, you will be led into an auditorium the size of Giants Stadium to be debriefed on the art of self-injection. If you're with a smaller practice, your class will be held in the "conference room," also known as the staff cafeteria. As you try to concentrate on the proper way to hold a subcutaneous needle, the office staff will be buzzing in and out, grabbing whipped yogurts and apples from the fridge. Either way, it's a traumatic experience; but as long as you leave the class with a basic understanding of how things work, along with detailed step-by-step instructions for home, you'll be fine.

Once you're comfortably settled into your classroom, there is the expected awkward period before things get started. You can cut the silence with a knife—that is, until your husband's Blackberry starts its familiar vibration buzz. It breaks the tension enough for a smirk here or there, but conversation is still taboo. There's an unspoken understanding—you're in a terrible place in your life, so is every-one else, why talk about it?

Finally, the nurse arrives and does her best to make the lecture interactive. She starts with the basics of human reproduction. A giant diagram of the female anatomy is rolled down from the ceiling like a projection screen, and she starts at the very beginning: "First a follicle begins to develop in the ovary," blah, blah, blah. At this point, you're confident you could teach a course on human reproduction at Columbia Medical School, and your silent mantra throughout her presentation is, "Come on, hurry up, get on with it." Your husband, on the other hand, is completely mesmerized by the presentation and all the "new" information. This just confirms he's been using the uh-huh nod on you all this time while all of your hard-earned research went in one ear and out the other.

Sex, Drugs and Rock 'n' Roll (Optional)

Doing her best to garner involvement, the nurse unexpectedly tosses out a question in the middle of her lecture: "Who can tell me what gonadotropins are?" There is a long, awkward silence. Your mind races like the avid board game lover you are. If this were Balderdash, you would blurt out the first definition that came to mind: "Some sort of fraternity trophy for the guy with the biggest gonads?" No. That can't be right. And this is no game, so you sit quietly and wait for someone else to speak up. No one does.

The nurse starts to draw the female anatomy on the whiteboard, and it becomes instantly obvious why she did not go to art school. Pointing to what you assume are the ovaries, the nurse explains that during a normal cycle, your body will produce one, maybe two eggs each month. When using gonadotropins, your body produces more follicles, each of which should include an egg; therefore, your odds of getting pregnant increase due to the greater number of eggs.

The nurse explains that the follicle stimulating hormone (FSH) is the magic ingredient in gonadotropins that make your ovaries work so hard to produce multiple eggs each cycle. When the nurse explains that FSH can be derived from either human proteins or synthetic materials, your mind starts to wander. Where the hell do "human proteins" come from? Sensing you're not the only one a bit confused, the nurse continues to explain that hFSH, human follicle stimulating hormone, is actually made from human urine. Gross!

Apparently the human-based gonadotropins also have small amounts of luteinizing hormone because it's difficult to completely filter out the LH. The "lab-created" gonadotropins, on the other hand, are pure FSH. The word "filter" sends your mind racing. Just where is all this urine coming from, and who's doing the filtering? Are unsuspecting visitors at Pfizer pharmaceutical stopping into the ladies room to relieve themselves while, unbeknownst to them, a giant labyrinth of urine collection devices are discreetly hidden in the plumbing?

There's probably a much more logical explanation. Maybe college students around the country are grabbing milk jugs and heading to the bathroom to collect their pee in exchange for five bucks. That's more than enough money to fund their festivities at dollar draft night. That theory gets tossed out the window when the nurse explains that hMGs (human menopausal gonadotropins) are actually made from the urine of postmenopausal women. Now your mind has gone from mug night to bingo night. Maybe it's better if you don't focus on how your medications came to be medications.

Now that you have a solid understanding of what drugs will be used, the nurse refers back to your ovaries on the whiteboard and brings the process to life by dotting in more and more eggs with her erasable pen. One word comes to mind: SEXTUPLETS. Your hand flies in the air. You've seen enough stories on *Dateline* to know you're not interested in converting your living room into a six-crib nursery with a rotating staff of volunteer nannies. When the nurse looks your way, you ask, "What are the risks of multiple births?"

"Good question," she replies. "According to the American Society for Reproductive Medicine, there is a significant increase in multiple pregnancies while taking gonadotropins. Without fertility drugs, multiple pregnancies only occur in 1 to 2 percent of the population. With gonadotropins, that number increases to approximately 20 percent. Most of those pregnancies are twins; however, triplets or more account for up to 5 percent of these multiple births."

You make a note to yourself: at your next appointment, you will ask your doctor specific questions about his philosophy on managing the risk of multiples and get some detailed information about his track record. The decision to work with a conservative doctor versus an aggressive one is a personal choice. While the conservative approach may not get the results as quickly, it will most likely save you from making the cover of *Time* magazine for setting the new record for live births in the United States.

Some more aggressive doctors have a single goal in mind: to get you pregnant . . . period. If they use an aggressive drug protocol and you end up with a high number of viable pregnancies, you may be forced to consider selective reduction. This is an extremely controversial subject and a decision no woman who is desperately trying to have a baby wants to face. But the fact remains: high-order multiple pregnancies pose a serious risk to both the babies and the mother. So before putting your trust and your health into your doctor's hands, have a candid conversation and take ownership of the process. Of course, you can't control everything, but aligning your expectations is a good first step.

The Risky Realities

The discussion around multiple pregnancies is the perfect segue to discuss the other risks associated with using gonadotropins. The nurse may hand out a neatly typed sheet of the potentially danger-ous side effects of taking gonadotropins and ask you to follow along as she walks through the risks. While the severest forms of these risks are unlikely, they are still possible and quite serious. So it is important that you weigh the information carefully before making a decision to proceed with the treatment.

Ovarian Hyperstimulation

Apparently there *can* be too much of a good thing. While the purpose of the gonadotropins is to get your body to produce more eggs than it would on its own, if your body produces too many, there can be serious consequences. Blood clots, kidney damage and ovarian twisting, as well as a buildup of fluid in the chest and abdomen, are a few of the dangers of ovarian hyperstimulation syndrome (OHSS). The most extreme cases may result in hospi-talization for weeks or longer, and surgery may be necessary to remove the fluid from the body, or, in the case of the ovarian twist-ing, the ovaries may need to be removed. Needless to say, OHSS is very serious and can be life threatening in its most severe form.

According to the American Society of Reproductive Medicine, severe OHSS occurs in only 1 percent of cases; however, a milder, non-life threatening reaction occurs in 10 to 20 percent of women using gonadotropins. These women experience bloating and dis-comfort, but typically the symptoms can be resolved without complications.

The best way to avoid OHSS, either moderate or severe, is through constant monitoring by your doctor. There's no way to predict how your body will react to the medication until you've actually started to use it. What may be a small dosage for one woman could wreak havoc on another. So your doctor will most likely start out conservatively, giving you a smaller dosage while he monitors your hormone levels via blood work and the number of follicles being produced with ultrasounds.

Typically, when using gonadotropins with IUI, you will begin taking your injections and go in for blood work and ultrasounds every two to three days while your follicles continue to grow and mature. Although you're certainly not thrilled with the thought of going in for blood and ultrasound tests every few days, now that you know the alternative, it seems reasonable.

Ectopic Pregnancy

Ectopic pregnancies, commonly known as tubal pregnancies, occur when the embryo attaches outside the uterus. While this occurs in only 1 percent of the normal population, the rates are slightly higher for women using gonadotropins.

When an embryo attaches in the fallopian tube, it doesn't have room to grow. If left undetected, it may actually burst through the fallopian tube and cause internal bleeding. One of our TTCs was so happy she was finally pregnant after months of treatment. Because she was pregnant with multiples, no one suspected another embryo could have possibly migrated north to implant. She experienced fatigue for several weeks but wrote it off to being pregnant. It wasn't until she got out of bed and collapsed on her way to the bathroom that she realized something was seriously wrong. It turned out she did have an ectopic pregnancy and had started to bleed internally. Luckily, she made it to the hospital in time, but she was not out of the woods until she had surgery and a blood transfusion.

Ovarian Cancer

The link between using fertility drugs and ovarian cancer has been widely reported and disputed between the medical community and the media. The official party line from the American Society of Reproductive Medicine is that the research studies to date have been inconclusive—there is no definitive proof fertility drugs do or do not cause ovarian cancer.

Apparently the chicken-and-egg theory is being investigated. Do infertility patients have some underlying condition that may contribute to their inability to get pregnant as well as increase their likelihood of developing cancer? The fact remains there are many unanswered questions about the connection between fertility drugs and cancer, especially the long-term effects of using the drugs. We recommend you do a little research yourself and address your concerns with your doctor. He should be able to point you to the most recent findings, so you can make an informed decision about whether you are comfortable proceeding with fertility drug usage.

Sign Here, Please

While your doctor's office will most likely emphasize the unlikelihood that you personally will fall subject to these catastrophic risks, they may ask you to sign a waiver at the end of the discussion. The waiver clearly states that you understand the cancer findings are inconclusive, and if research should surface at some point in the future proving fertility drugs do in fact cause cancer, you will not hold the doctor liable. Yes, we live in a litigious society, but signing on the dotted line puts the severity of the situation in focus. The decision should not be taken lightly. Sit down with your husband and have a serious conversation about what risks you are willing and unwilling to take to build your family.

The ART of Injections

We think ART is the perfect acronym for assisted reproductive technology. While the term "assisted reproductive technology" captures the medical sensibility, the acronym "ART" speaks to the goal—creating the ultimate work of art: a new life.

Rather than picking up a palette and a paintbrush, you are handed a 27-gauge needle and a syringe to learn the art of the subcutaneous injection. You may ask yourself why this medication has to be given through an injection. Why not a pill? We guarantee that if men were the primary target of fertility treatments, gonadotropins would be available in a fast-acting nasal spray. How is it possible a tiny pill like Viagra comes with a warning that it could cause a four-hour erection in the senior-citizen set, but it takes a series of painful shots to jump-start the fertile feminine you?

In answer to this question, your doctor explains that the potency of these drugs is not diluted in shot form because they do not have to be processed through your body's digestive system. That makes sense until you think back to your aging grandparents and the vast array of ailments they somehow managed to fight off with a fistful of pills. "Honey, can you hand me my pillbox from the counter?" they would ask when you were spending the night away from home at Hotel Granny. "Pillbox" was the understatement of the century. It was a giant plastic container with seven individual lids labeled Monday through Sunday. Like a Christmas Advent calendar, each lid was lifted to unveil each day's medicinal treats. Treatments for high blood pressure, heart conditions, bad cholesterol—you name it, the pillbox had it. But somehow, your grandparent's medication miraculously managed to maintain its potency, even though it had to make its way down an eighty-year-old esophagus with a refreshing lemonade chaser.

Even if you were the captain of the college debate team, there's really no need to voice your well-thought-out argument against the validity of injectable versus oral medications. Gonadotropins don't come in pill form, so accept it and move on.

Learning the Lingo

Before you get to the good part of the class, where the big shiny needle gets shoved into your hypothetical ass, you must first learn some basic medical terminology.

First, you learn the two types of injections. There are subcutaneous, meaning the injection is given just under the skin, and there are intramuscular, which means the medicine must be injected directly into the muscle tissue. We like to refer to these two types of shots as "Ouch" and "Holy Shit!" respectively.

Next, you must become familiar with fertility math. The medications can be measured in two ways, either international units (IUs) or ampules (amps). Why isn't there one consistent form of measurement? We have no idea. Maybe it's like the big push in the 1970s for the United States to join the rest of the world by putting down the yardstick and picking up the meter stick. Great intention; it just never happened—the foot-long hotdog lives and so do amps and IUs.

The good news is the conversion from amps to IUs is much easier than trying to remember that there are 25.4 millimeters in 1 inch. Just remember, 1 amp equals 75 IUs. So if your doctor calls and says, "Take 2 amps of Gonal-F, and call me in the morning," simply measure 150 IUs, and you're done.

Once you have the measurements down, you will learn how to mix the medications. Most of these meds come in powder form, along with a container of bacteriostatic water. You should use only this water for mixing your medications. If something happens and you drop, spill or lose your bacteriostatic water, don't run over to the tap and fill her up. In the injections class, you'll learn how much water to mix in, how to extract the medication and how to make sure all of the air bubbles are out of the syringe. In some cases, multiple medications can be given together, which is very good news because it means one less poke for you.

Once you have all the measuring and mixing mastered, it's time to move on to the intimidating part—the injection.

The Ouch Shot

The nurse pulls out a subcutaneous needle and tries to lessen the impact by announcing this is the same type of needle diabetics use every day to give themselves insulin. Of course, you feel terrible for the diabetics of the world, but it doesn't make it any easier as you look at the needle and envision where it's headed.

The subcutaneous needle is extremely thin and measures approximately one-half inch long; that's smaller than the length of your thumbnail (unless you have very small thumbs). But still, it's sharp and scary.

Handing out the sample needles in class is like handing a pack of matches to a bunch of fifth graders. Even though you are told to wait until the instructions are given, everyone instantly starts fidgeting with the needles. The nurse tells you the first thing you must do is gently wiggle the protective needle cap back and forth to remove it. The cap is secured tightly for safety reasons, and if you use brute force to pull it off, your hand may recoil when it finally breaks free, and you'll end up stabbing yourself. She no sooner says this than someone in the class lets out a yelp and holds out her blood-pulsing thumb. With an "I told you so" look on her face, the nurse announces the class will take a short break while she bandages up the first victim.

Once everyone settles down, it's time to get started again. Most subcutaneous shots are given in the lower abdomen below the belly button or in the outer side of the upper thigh. You must be able to pinch an inch of skin to give the shot, and according to the nurse, everyone, regardless of their weight, can find an inch to pinch. For the first time in your life, you're happy you indulged in a doughnut from time to time, but as you look across the room at a supermodel-skinny woman, you wonder where the hell her shot is going. She couldn't possibly pinch a millimeter, never mind an inch.

In class, you will practice giving the injections on a gelatinous ball, which unfortunately closely resembles the consistency of your lower abdomen. First step, clean the skin with an alcohol swab. Don't blow on the area to hurry things along; you'll just add more germs. When the area is dry, the shot-giver removes the cap from the needle, pinches an inch of skin and injects the needle at a forty-five-degree angle. Once the needle is all the way in, you press the plunger until it won't go any further, release the skin and pull the needle out. If there's any blood at the injection site, apply pressure with a cotton ball for a minute or until the bleeding stops.

Needles cannot be randomly tossed in the trash once you're done. They are medical waste and must be discarded properly; otherwise, they will eventually wash up on the Jersey Shore and ruin the summer for everyone. Your doctor's office will tell you to designate a puncture-proof container for needles, for example, a coffee can or a heavy-duty laundry detergent bottle. When the container is full, take it to the doctor's office, where they will dispose of it according to regulated guidelines.

The Holy Shit Shot

Unlike the subcutaneous needle, the nurse does not hand out a sample of the intramuscular (IM) needles; rather, she insists you follow along with her until she has covered all the instructions. The reason for this is obvious the moment she wiggles free the protective plastic cap to reveal the notorious needle. While the subcutaneous needles are barely the size of your thumbnail, the intramuscular needles are as big as your thumb! Measuring an inch and a half long, they bring a gasp from everyone in the room— those giving as well as those receiving the shots. When you glance over at the profile of the super skinny girl, you think the needle may be just long enough that, regardless of where she sticks it, odds are it's going to poke through the other side.

If you have the slightest fear of needles, you will feel a wave of panic rush over you like you've never experienced before. The nurse tries to tell you it isn't as bad as it looks and explains that some of you may have already experienced this needle when receiving the hCG trigger shot. Even if you have, there's a big difference between getting the shot at the doctor's office and having your nervous husband's trembling hands try to give you one at home.

Because the intramuscular shot must be given directly into muscle tissue, the location of the shot is pretty much set. You guessed it . . . the gluteus maximus, the bum, the buttocks, the derriere, the behind. Call it what you want, that giant needle is headed for your ass.

Unless you have buns of steel, you can't just stick the needle anywhere in your bum and hope to hit muscle. You need a plan. If you divide each "cheek" into four equal-size quadrants, you want the upper outer box—in other words, the fleshy part to the side of your hip bone. If you're a bit overwhelmed by choosing the right spot, you may opt to have the nurse draw a bull's-eye on your buttocks to leave nothing to chance. Not a bad idea, just make sure it's not bikini season, or you'll be the talk of the town.

The actual steps of an IM injection are basically the same as a subcutaneous shot. First, clean the area, then gently squeeze the muscle and finally insert the needle, but this time at a ninety-degree angle. Once the needle is all the way in, pull back on the plunger to make sure you haven't hit a blood vessel. If you do hit a blood vessel you'll see blood in the vial. Take a deep breath and remove the needle. Replace it with a clean needle and try again. When all is clear, push the plunger down until all the medication has been injected, release the skin, remove the needle and throw it away in the "sharps" container.

The good news is (and we use the word "good" loosely), most of the medications you'll be using for the IUI cycle can be given with the subcutaneous needle, so you should be spared the torture of the IM shot. Your doctor may prescribe an IM needle with hCG. However, for IUI patients, this shot can also be given subcutaneously, so make sure you speak up and request the smaller needle.

The First Night

To:	Courtney <Courtney@conceptionchronicles.com>; Shelly <Shelly@conceptionchronicles.com>
From:	Patty <Patty@conceptionchronicles.com>
Subject:	**About Last Night**

Well girls, we did it. I took my first fertility shot last night.

It was a lot harder than I thought. I had on a brave face for most of the day, although I was completely dreading it, and there wasn't a minute it wasn't on my mind. When it came time to get everything ready, Scott and I broke out the directions and carefully mixed all the medication. I was lying on the bed, trying to psyche myself up, but the minute Scott said, "Are you ready?" I burst into tears. He felt so bad and just kept hugging me tighter and tighter telling me he was so sorry I had to go through this.

I can't believe it's come to this. By the time I finally regained my composure, the tension was pretty high. When Scott pinched my stomach to prepare for the shot, I flinched, felt the needle go in and let out an overly dramatic "OUCH!"

He had the funniest look on his face. When I told him how much it hurt, he confessed he hadn't actually given me the shot. Apparently when I flinched, I bumped his arm, and he accidentally stuck me. He wasn't ready, so when I screamed, he instinctively pulled the needle out without pushing down the plunger. We had to do it all over again.

Believe it or not, we actually laughed! Start to finish, the process took us over an hour, but we got it done. I've got to believe this is going to get better.

To: Patty <Patty@conceptionchronicles.com>
From: Shelly <Shelly@conceptionchronicles.com>
Cc: Courtney <Courtney@conceptionchronicles.com>
Subject: **RE: About Last Night**

I'm so proud of you. I promise I'll never complain about sex on demand again. I'm sure it's only going to get better for you from here. Hang in there.

To: Patty <Patty@conceptionchronicles.com>
From: Courtney <Courtney@conceptionchronicles.com>
CC: Shelly <Shelly@conceptionchronicles.com>
Subject: **RE: RE: About Last Night**

How many more days of this do you have left? For every day you get through it, you should treat yourself (and Scott) to something nice. Stay strong, my little friend.

Like every other terrifying experience in life—giving a presentation to a room full of people, going to the dentist for a root canal or interviewing for a job you really want—it's often the buildup that is far worse than the actual event. The same is true for the first night of your injections. The anticipation leading up to the first time the sharp little subcutaneous needle meets your skin is almost unbearable. But once you've actually done it a few times, you realize it's not nearly as bad as you thought.

Once you start down the road of injections, you may feel another slight shift in your relationship, only this time it's for the better. While your husband had a nonspeaking role in the *Clomid Masterpiece Theater*—his job was to simply hand off his sample as he headed out the door—he is now featured center stage for the production of *Injections*. Unless you take on the burden of giving the shots to yourself, your husband will now experience first hand the stress and anxiety surrounding your treatment. If it turns out your husband hates needles more than you do, this step may be even more traumatic for him than for you.

Either way, you reconnect and on some level realize you are the only two people in the world who understand the enormity of what you are going through. Of course, you may have girlfriends who have been through it, but this is your life, and the personal implications of the treatment's success or failure will impact you and your husband forever. You may find that you start to cling to each other a little more than usual since you are both finally feeling the same way.

Becoming a Pro

Remember the good old days when the words, "It's your turn to get the shots," meant fighting the crowd on dollar shooter night only to return thirty minutes later with a tray full of kamikazes for you and your friends? Welcome to the new you. Those same words have a drastically different meaning. Now it's a point of negotiation as to who is going to leave the couch in the middle of the movie to prepare the medication. The drama surrounding the shot is gone; now it's just a matter of inconvenience. We have friends who became so comfortable with the process, they could mix the medication and give themselves the shot all while talking with the phone cradled on their shoulder.

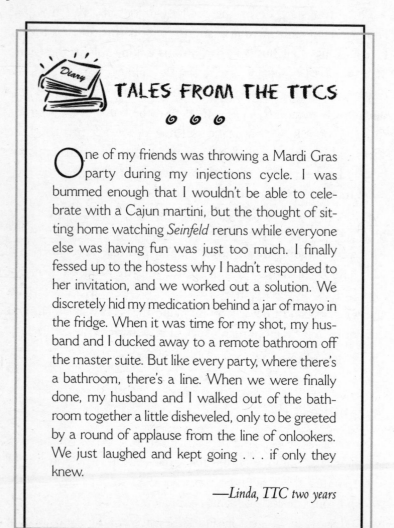

TALES FROM THE TTCS

ne of my friends was throwing a Mardi Gras party during my injections cycle. I was bummed enough that I wouldn't be able to celebrate with a Cajun martini, but the thought of sitting home watching *Seinfeld* reruns while everyone else was having fun was just too much. I finally fessed up to the hostess why I hadn't responded to her invitation, and we worked out a solution. We discretely hid my medication behind a jar of mayo in the fridge. When it was time for my shot, my husband and I ducked away to a remote bathroom off the master suite. But like every party, where there's a bathroom, there's a line. When we were finally done, my husband and I walked out of the bathroom together a little disheveled, only to be greeted by a round of applause from the line of onlookers. We just laughed and kept going . . . if only they knew.

—*Linda, TTC two years*

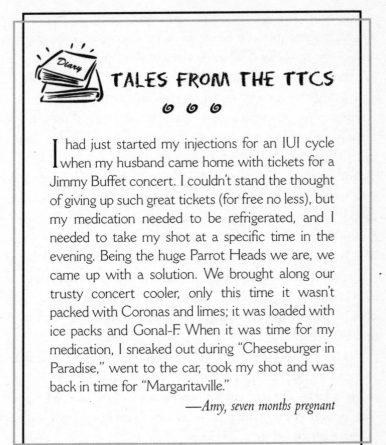

TALES FROM THE TTCS

I had just started my injections for an IUI cycle when my husband came home with tickets for a Jimmy Buffet concert. I couldn't stand the thought of giving up such great tickets (for free no less), but my medication needed to be refrigerated, and I needed to take my shot at a specific time in the evening. Being the huge Parrot Heads we are, we came up with a solution. We brought along our trusty concert cooler, only this time it wasn't packed with Coronas and limes; it was loaded with ice packs and Gonal-F. When it was time for my medication, I sneaked out during "Cheeseburger in Paradise," went to the car, took my shot and was back in time for "Margaritaville."

—*Amy, seven months pregnant*

Let the Games Begin

The stakes for each month's efforts are even higher now that you are using injectables. Of course, you never thought you'd be in a place where sex was a backup for making a baby. But you are. You know the IUI will be perfectly timed, and this month you're actually having two IUIs on separate days to cover your bases. Still, you don't want to leave anything to chance, so you maintain the sex-on-demand ritual.

You remember the disturbing side effects discussed in class, but you don't remember anyone mentioning your stomach would blow up like the Michelin Man a few days into the process. It's not like you had six-pack abs before, but now the squishy factor is off the charts. This is certainly not how a girl wants to feel when she is gearing up for an evening of seduction, but you gotta' work with what you have. The skimpy sexsuit is now replaced with a flowing silk nightie, circa 1950. At least it's not boxers.

And so this is your life . . . shot, sex, blood work, ultrasound; shot, sex, blood work, ultrasound; shot, sex, blood work, ultrasound. Until one day, your doctor calls to say everything looks great—your follicles are mature and ready to go. He tells you to take your trigger shot that evening, abstain from sexual relations and come in the next morning for insemination. Once the insemination is over, you're done. No more shots, no more running to the doctor's office every two days for blood work. Now, it's back to the dreaded 2ww.

When you call your husband and fill him in on what will and will not be happening later in the evening, he replies, "I never thought I'd see the day, but I'm sick of sex." You're both relieved it's over, or almost over, and you spend a quiet evening at home allowing yourself to dream once again.

chapter eleven

What Do You Tell the Paparazzi?

Thursday	Notes
	- Happy hr. w/ work-call to cancel!

Friday	Notes	Saturday	Notes
- ~~Dinner w/ Mike & Mary~~		- ~~Baby shower for Amy~~	

You've made a crucial mistake. In a weak moment, you decide to share your fertility hysteria with a friend. Unfortunately, history has shown this is not necessarily the friend who is willing to keep your secrets. You swore to yourself (and to your husband) you would keep the most intimate details of your pregnancy struggles limited to your closest girlfriends. And now this. The friend most likely to pen the neighborhood edition of *The National Enquirer* is suddenly privy to your most personal particulars.

How did it happen? Your friend may have innocently asked how "things" were going, and on this particular day, "things" were looking pretty good. So, caught up in the possibility of what could be, you share your excitement with her. You tell her this might finally be "the month" after so many months of trying. Before you know it, you've taken her blow-by-blow through your fertility journey, leaving not a morsel of detail left to her imagination.

Or perhaps you were completely caught off guard one day at the office by a newly pregnant coworker, who unflinchingly commanded, "You better get pregnant soon, so I have someone to shop with for maternity clothes." Since it's never been your natural inclination to lie, you instead revert to insane, over-the-top honesty and confess you have just started your second cycle of injectables. Not only does she have a million follow-up questions, which she fires at you with the zeal of a DA, she also insinuates that your later-in-life approach to having a family might be the problem. You want to tell her you've actually been trying for quite a while or you don't really consider yourself to be approaching your golden years, but you decide to just keep your mouth shut. It's not really any of her business, and she probably wouldn't listen anyway.

Unguarded and vulnerable, you've given away too much. The consequence: prepare yourself for anything. From this day forward, you may be inundated with questions you never thought you would have to answer from anyone other than your husband or doctor.

Did you get your period? When are you ovulating? Have you thought about Clomid, injections, IVF? Your return from an innocent trip to the dry cleaners is met with a phone call from the nice, but now noticeably nosy, neighbor across the street. You ran into her last week after a disappointing doctor's appointment and somehow ended up spilling your guts to her about everything—the injections, IUI, the full monty. You knew it was probably a mistake to confide in her, but she was so sweet and seemed genuinely interested, and at the time, you just needed to talk to someone. Well, you were right—it was a big-time blunder. She's now just another person who knows way too much and wants to know even more. Today, her questions don't feel remotely supportive but driven out of cunning curiosity, like she's writing a book. "Was your IUI today? How did it go? Did it hurt? How long did it take? Did your husband go with you?" You wish she'd leave this chapter out.

No matter how it comes out, you immediately regret opening up and wish you could take it all back. Unfortunately, it's too late. Now you'll spend the next several weeks wondering who knows what and which dinner parties will be serving up your fertility issues along with grilled salmon, rice pilaf and a healthy portion of pity. After discussing your paranoia with your husband, you mutually agree to decline all dinner invitations for the next few months.

The Paparazzi

To make matters worse, people are coming out of the woodwork and starting to ask some very candid questions. Remember back at Thanksgiving when you jokingly revealed to your curious gaggle of aunts that you and the hubby had pulled the goalie? Or last spring when you began openly asking every mother you knew for baby-making advice? Well, a year has gone by, and they haven't received a birth announcement, so the tables have turned, and you are considered fair game. Some may be discreet with their questions, while others come right out and ask if you are having marital problems.

The paparazzi appear where and when you least expect them. What's incredible is it doesn't really matter if you've ever broached the subject of children with them. You may have never even discussed *anything* remotely personal, but for some inexplicable reason, they feel justified to ask you just about anything as well as to offer their unsolicited advice on all things baby.

It's All Relative

One of our TTCs received an unbelievable call one rainy Sunday afternoon from an aunt on her husband's side of the family. For the record, our TTC and this in-law had never had a conversation about anything more personal than discussing if they preferred Reddiwip or Cool Whip on their holiday pumpkin pie. The phone call was literally the first one the relative had made to our TTC in the five years they had been "family." There'd been no birthday cards exchanged, no "joke" e-mails forwarded to one another, no periodic checking-in to see how things were going.

Needless to say, our TTC was beyond curious when her caller ID flashed seven unfamiliar digits following the area code usually paired with her in-law's number. After the obligatory, "Hello. How are you?" the aunt hastily transitioned to the obvious point of her call. "I was just reading an article about older couples who can't have kids, and I thought of you. It tells you everything you need to know about adoption. How to start the whole process. It has Web sites and phone numbers of government agencies you can contact. Literally, everything." Our TTC was astounded and appalled and barely uttered the words, "Thank you, but we haven't really considered adoption." For some bizarre reason, our TTC felt the need to be both polite and gracious to a woman who was shamelessly stepping over the line. Despite our TTC's reply, the aunt dismissively said she would pop the article in the mail and hung up. The call was over as quickly as it had begun.

In reality, our TTC had just begun her fertility workup and had no real idea of what lay ahead for her and her husband. Not that it mattered—clearly the family was three steps ahead of them. While our TTC's biggest concern was wondering if and when she was ovulating, apparently the in-laws had completely written off her ability to give birth.

The Whole Truth and Nothing but the Truth

To:	Courtney <Courtney@conceptionchronicles.com>; Shelly <Shelly@conceptionchronicles.com>
From:	Patty <Patty@conceptionchronicles.com>
Subject:	**Blabbermouth**

I had breakfast with my old boss this morning—we get together every few months just to catch up. While I was devouring my omelet, he flat out asked me if Scott and I were going to have kids. I'm sure he was just asking to be polite, but all of sudden I started pouring out my heart. I have no idea what came over me—I haven't even told some of my closest friends what we're going through.

I'm sure my half-hour fertility monologue wasn't what he was expecting, but he couldn't have been nicer. It turned out he had a close friend who had been through the same thing, so he completely understood how hard it's been.

To: Patty <Patty@conceptionchronicles.com>
From: Shelly <Shelly@conceptionchronicles.com>
Cc: Courtney <Courtney@conceptionchronicles.com>
Subject: **RE: Blabbermouth**

It's nice to see you can find some support where you least expect it. I'm so sick of everyone asking me when we're going to have #2. I just avoid the topic all together.

What is it that forces your hand into telling the paparazzi more than you really want or prevents you from responding in a manner that allows you to remain in control of the conversation? Most of us are not naturally deceitful, but you wish you could keep the information download on your own terms. Yet when asked frankly about your plans to have children, there is usually an overwhelming feeling of obligation to tell the truth, the whole truth and not just a watered-down version of it. The truth seems to pour out of you like an overflowing bathtub, although you had no intention of revealing even the most insignificant of details. Maybe it's as simple as you've never been a good liar and don't feel you can fabricate an explanation with any real conviction. But there is also just something innately uncomfortable about lying to your friends and family about the efforts you are taking to have a baby.

Okay, so it's not exactly easy to put off sincere interest from your close friends and family, but what do you do when the questions feel especially invasive, unwarranted or don't seem to have the slightest hint of good intentions behind them? We've come up with a handy list of ten answers that are certain to stop the maddening, meddling, over-the-top paparazzi dead in their tracks. These are surefire inquisition-enders, and the silence that ensues will give you plenty of time to elude the awkward moment that's sure to follow, not to mention the satisfaction you'll have leaving your listener with his or her jaw dropped opened.

The questions may seem innocent upon first reading them, and if they are coming from someone who really cares about you, then they probably are. But you'll also know when there's something not so nice hidden behind the words. Carry the answers with you like your AAA card—you never know when you'll need them.

QUESTIONS: Are you going to have kids? When are you going to have kids? Do you want kids? Do you want more kids?

ANSWERS:

1. We can't. I'm barren.
2. It's not likely. My husband suffers from erectile dysfunction. (*Optional:* Add "hereditary" when asked by a particularly nosy in-law.)
3. We're getting a boat instead. It's way more fun.
4. Our dog (cat, pig, bird) is our baby. And he's much less of a hassle than a kid. The best part is, we can board him for only ten bucks a night whenever we want to get away.
5. We're going to start trying as soon as our couple's therapist says it's okay.
6. I actually despise children.
7. We're going to start trying as soon as I stop taking antidepressants.
8. No, I like to sleep too much. I would never want to deal with the 2 A.M. feedings.

9. I'm not sure we'd be good parents. We have a standing reservation for Friday night happy hour, not to mention Saturday morning Bloody Marys. A hangover is bad enough without some baby screaming.
10. We wanted to until we spent time with your kids.

BONUS ANSWER:

11. It's none of your f—ing business.

When You Just Can't Help Yourself

If the above answers don't work for you (and we agree there are probably few situations where they are appropriate or warranted, although they would be fun to deliver, wouldn't they?), then what do you do about talking too much? When you were taking Clomid like baby aspirin and zipping off to the YMCA after your IUIs, you felt comfortable talking about your fertility anguish with your girlfriends at the gym. You had no problem, in between squats and lunges, reporting on the number of follicles you produced in a given cycle. Bicep curls gave way to conversations about hot flashes and the quality of your husband's sperm. You could toss out comments like, "Hmmm, if I had to do IVF, I suppose I would," but you never really believed it would come to that. Guess what? It has.

Whether it's bad news you receive after a laparoscopy or your third strike at injections/IUI, all point to the same, much more serious conclusions and choices you will now have to make: IVF, adoption, surrogacy, egg donor or possibly even an embryo donor. These are not topics you want to discuss during a scheduled spin class.

Unfortunately, you have opened the door, unleashed the beast, let the colossal cat out of the bag. The point is, you have fully exposed yourself and don't quite know how to reel back in the fertility hotline. You find yourself trying to cope with your intensifying fertility circumstances while answering questions that, quite frankly, you yourself are not comfortable with yet. You try to ward off unwanted comments but find yourself trapped in situations that won't allow it. Conversations with friends are no longer sprinkled with periodic queries; instead, they are now a full interrogation about your fertility problems. Once again, you are sputtering out the truth.

We have TTCs who simply cannot stop themselves from answering a fertility question with complete honesty. Not because they have lofty moral principles, but because they are so unprepared to fend off a straightforward inquiry like, "Have you gotten your blood test back to find out if you are pregnant?" Before they know it, they've blurted out that their doctor just called to say it was negative and they will probably have to start IVF next month. Amazingly, the TTC's husband is not the first to know—again. We're not certain if our fertility doctor is secretly slipping us "truth serum" every time we visit his clinic, but for those of us struggling along the path, we find we just can't help but tell the truth.

Our suggestion is to try to take time with your husband to sort through your ever-changing situation. When it comes to topics like IVF or other ART techniques, be comfortable with your decisions well before discussing them with others, and try to prepare answers that will allow you some latitude as well as the option to change your mind without having to explain yourself.

And remember, you are not required to purge your soul no matter who's doing the asking. If someone happens to probe with a question as personal as, "When do you think you'll be doing IVF?" instead of offering the details of the very private conversation you had with your husband last night, you may reply with, "We haven't really made any decisions. We're going to give ourselves a break for the next few months." This should halt any further questioning and also allow you the opportunity to steal back some of your precious hijacked privacy.

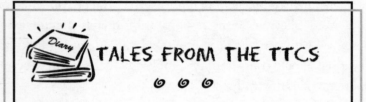

TALES FROM THE TTCS

𝟞 𝟞 𝟞

After my second cycle of injections, I became pregnant with twins. My fertility saga had gone on for so long, I'd eventually shared all the details of my treatments and subsequent pregnancy with all my friends and most of my acquaintances. My greatest fear was realized at birth, when only one of the babies, my daughter, survived. After months of trying to recover from the depths of despair I felt after losing my other child, my first night out was attending a dinner party at the home of a close friend.

While heading to the restroom, I walked by a small circle of women who were chatting away. I knew I would likely be a topic of hushed conversation after experiencing what I had, but I never imagined how cruel some people could be at the expense of someone's heartrending loss. As I made my way to the loo, I overheard one woman saying quietly to the rest of the group, "Well, what did she expect would happen taking all of those fertility drugs?"

Needless to say, by the time I reached the bathroom, I was in tears. I spent the next ten minutes trying to regain my composure while reminding myself over and over again that all I ever wanted to be was a mother and that I'd made responsible decisions in order to get pregnant and give birth to my daughter.

—*Maggie, mother of one*

Warning: Paparazzi May Be Closer Than They Appear

The only thing worse than getting the third degree from your friends is your mother-in-law wondering out loud when she's going to be a grandmother. Another TTC we know has a mother-in-law who kept a two-inch gap on her "grandmother's charm bracelet" reserved for the sterling silver silhouette of the grandchild her son and daughter-in-law had yet to deliver. Each and every family gathering included an uncalled-for remark akin to, "I've still got room on this bracelet for at least one more. When are you two going to make me a grandma again?"

Mothers-in-law can be especially clueless as to the damage their speculations can cause. Her "innocent" comments may also feature well-seasoned sarcasm as she implies you have made a conscious decision not to have children because of your "fill in the blank"— age, career, selfishness, desire to travel or wish to save more money or buy a bigger house. Maybe you did put off having kids based on one of the above, or maybe you just weren't ready until now. No matter what the reason, it's really no one's place to point the finger or pass judgment on your decisions. Hopefully, you can find a gentle way to let her know the not-so-subtle hinting and the outright ribbing are making it harder on you than she probably even realizes. If not, humor usually works better (as does merlot) than letting it come between you and your husband.

The Mother of All Paparazzi: Dear Old Mom

Can your own mother really be considered paparazzi? Well, if the snoop fits. It may not be easy to figure out exactly where your mother is coming from or what's really on her mind when discussing your baby-making issues. Her unpredictable reactions to your fertility struggles have left you wondering if she is quietly cheering you on or if she just wishes you'd give up. For someone who'd always dreamed out loud about becoming a grandmother someday, she now has you completely confused.

During your weekly call she's more than excited to talk endlessly about the new handbag she bought to match the floral dress she purchased for your cousin's wedding. However, the second the conversation lulls and you bring up your most recent doctor's visit, she seems to slip into a funk. Sure, she makes the requisite inquiry each call, "How you are feeling, dear?" or "How are *things* going?" but with each question, you hear her inhale then hold her breath while she waits for you to answer. Is she worried she won't have helpful motherly advice to share, or is she seriously concerned for your mental and physical health? Probably a mixture of both.

Trying to decipher what your mother's reaction will be each time you talk to her about your fertility problems is like playing poker and queens are wild. You may think you know what you have in your hand, and then you're dealt a lady, and everything instantly changes. So don't bet on your mom reacting the same way each time—she may surprise you.

To:	Shelly <Shelly@conceptionchronicles.com>;
	Courtney <Courtney@conceptionchronicles.com>
From:	Patty <Patty@conceptionchronicles.com>
Subject:	**She's come a long way, baby**

Considering my mom was skeptical (to say the least) about my temperature charting, it's amazing she's been so supportive about the high-tech treatment we're considering. I always knew she'd be there for me, but she's completely outdone herself. It's so comforting to have her in my corner—unconditionally.

To:	Patty <Patty@conceptionchronicles.com>
From:	Courtney <Courtney@conceptionchronicles.com>
Cc:	Shelly <Shelly@conceptionchronicles.com>
Subject:	**RE: She's come a long way, baby**

I know how much it means to have your mom's support. No one can make you feel better in tough times.

Before you pour your heart out and stand with open arms waiting for your mother's loving embrace, remember that she's a wild card. Mothers who have been cheering you on with the enthusiasm of a Little League parent so far may suddenly take a turn when the stakes are raised. When you told your mom you were taking Clomid, she said, "Good for you," and continued the conversation. But when you announced you were thinking about IVF, the chatter stopped dead in its tracks. Thinking she just needed a minute to collect her thoughts, you asked if she was still there. After clearing her throat, she said, "Honey, maybe it's time to give up and move on." This certainly wasn't the response you expected or hoped for, and suddenly you were the one with nothing to say.

Today's world of fertility treatment is like having a baby in outer space as far as your mom is concerned, so you have to give her a bit of a break if it takes her a while to soak it all in. She may have preconceived notions about assisted reproduction and may need some time to reconfigure what she understands and believes now that her own daughter is faced with some very difficult and life-altering decisions.

There is one thing your mother will be certain of today, tomorrow and the next day—the more serious and invasive the treatment may be, the more she will worry about the effects it will have on her baby. As you sort through your conversations with your mom, you begin to realize, "I'm her child, and she's concerned about me and my well-being. She'd rather see me healthy and happy than struggling with fertility imperfection. She is, after all, a mother at heart. She is my mom, and she loves me."

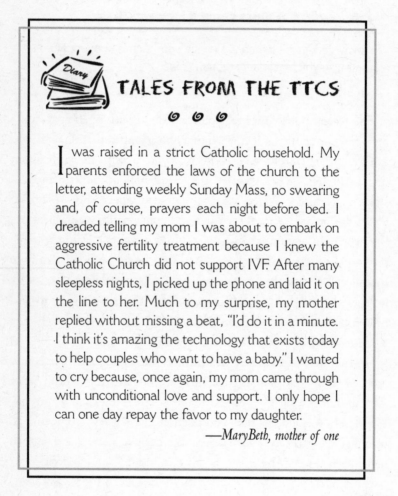

TALES FROM THE TTCS

I was raised in a strict Catholic household. My parents enforced the laws of the church to the letter, attending weekly Sunday Mass, no swearing and, of course, prayers each night before bed. I dreaded telling my mom I was about to embark on aggressive fertility treatment because I knew the Catholic Church did not support IVF. After many sleepless nights, I picked up the phone and laid it on the line to her. Much to my surprise, my mother replied without missing a beat, "I'd do it in a minute. I think it's amazing the technology that exists today to help couples who want to have a baby." I wanted to cry because, once again, my mom came through with unconditional love and support. I only hope I can one day repay the favor to my daughter.

—*MaryBeth, mother of one*

Mrs. Clean Is Mean

Don't be surprised if the paparazzi also come disguised as unsuspecting household help. You realize you are safe from no one when your cleaning lady one day declares, "You better hurry up if you want to have kids. You're getting old." These words amaze you not only for their sheer boldness but also for the clarity in which she delivers them. After three years of struggling to communicate through broken English and wild hand gestures that you do not want her to use furniture polish on your antique armoire, she suddenly has a Ph.D. in human reproduction and not a trace of an accent.

Yes, you fire Dora. After years of subpar cleaning and an irremovable waxy buildup on Grandma's mahogany wardrobe, you have finally had enough and decide to let her go. Of course, it had absolutely nothing to do with her insult.

Paparazzi by Day, Fertility Expert by Night

On slow nights, the paparazzi also double as authorities in the fertility field. Again, no matter if they've never personally experienced trouble getting pregnant, much like our fertile friend "The Professor," the paparazzi have an answer for any and every problem they are certain you have. Maybe they've read about the latest fertility treatments in a women's magazine or overheard a conversation about a laparoscopy at the hair salon; they have no qualms passing on medical advice with all of the confidence of a trained specialist.

During a phone call one night, a TTC was tiptoeing around the details of her escalating fertility treatment with a friend who had been less than sensitive about our TTC's pregnancy challenges. While trying to keep her friend in the loop but without revealing too much detail, our TTC was cut off midsentence with, "You know, you really don't have a lot of time to mess around." Mess around? Who was she to judge our TTC's efforts as lacking urgency? Our TTC was both angry and disappointed her friend would so easily criticize her when all she was trying to do was keep the doors of communication open yet still maintain some small sense of privacy.

Cruel Irony

You've learned the hard way that sharing everything with everyone is not the smartest thing to do when you are trying to get pregnant. But what do you do when you finally have the ultimate good news to share? You are finally pregnant and cannot possibly keep it to yourself! After sharing the elation with your husband, your first inclination might be to sprint to the phone and call everyone you know so you can share your wonderful news.

Don't do it! Yes, it will be excruciating to refrain from hitting every number programmed into your speed dial, but we strongly suggest you take a moment and remind yourself that, technically, you have been pregnant only a few days. It's tempting to call all the people who asked month after month if you were pregnant, those same people who charted your cycle with you and knew better than your husband your exact ovulation day. But there's a good reason for the standard three-month wait couples employ before blasting the news to the masses; sadly, miscarriages are very common in the first trimester of pregnancy. So before you spread the word of your happy news, think about how uncomfortable you would be telling the paparazzi if the unspeakable happens.

We send this caution because if you do, regrettably, miscarry, you will feel like the entire world is crumbling around you. It will be difficult to face your closest supporters with the news, never mind the neighbor down the street. Uttering the words, "I miscarried," is equally as heartbreaking as expressing the words, "I'm pregnant," is blissful.

Whether it's six, ten or twenty weeks into your pregnancy, your heart will break at the loss of what will never be. The sorrow will stick with you, but it's the irony of the situation that stings the most. You struggled for months, maybe years, to conceive, and when you finally felt the joy of being pregnant, it was ripped away from you so quickly. It's a cruel twist of fate. A small voice in the back of your mind may have been telling you something just wasn't right, but you attributed your worries to the many defenses you'd perfected along the fertility path. You know miscarriages happen, but you still ask, "Why me?"

Couple this gut-wrenching event with the series of phone calls that are sure to come from the lot of friends and acquaintances you let know about the pregnancy and the experience is more than unbearable. Suggestions on how to reduce morning sickness are replaced with, "I'm so sorry, but it was for the best." The best for whom? You wonder as you hang up the phone and dive under the covers in an effort to avoid any more unsolicited, useless sympathy. Women who have never experienced a miscarriage will quickly tell you that it happens more than you realize, and you'll be pregnant again before you know it. You think to yourself, "But I don't want to be pregnant *again*. I want to be pregnant now, with this baby. I wanted this one."

The Scarlet "I"

Are most of your friends married with children? Is a fun Saturday night getting together and letting the kids play in the basement? Has "wine" been replaced by the "whine" of a two-year-old at most of the parties you attend? Do you find half-eaten tortilla chips floating in the salsa? Are juice boxes and bottles of water filling the coolers once packed with ice-cold beer? If you answered "yes" to any of these questions, then chances are you may eventually face another wonderful by-product of prolonged infertility—fallout in your social life.

Being the fun-loving couple you are, your names may have always topped the invitation list when it came to friends and family. But the longer you try and are unsuccessful at getting pregnant, the more uncomfortable social situations may become for everyone—

especially if children play a starring role in the festivities.

Overnight, it seems like your mailbox is filled with invitations to celebrate new births and observe religious rites of passage or maybe it's to enjoy birthday cake and a friendly game of Pin the Tail on the Donkey while cowboys and princesses fight over who gets to go first. If you happen to be the only couple in your group without kids or you are not "expecting," these events can become more and more awkward over time for you and your hosts. You may have always been known by all of the kids as the couple who gave great presents, but their parents may stop including you at the festivities if they think they are sparing you from enduring increasingly difficult situations.

This is where it gets tricky—they're right. You don't want to miss the christenings, baby namings or first birthdays; they are important milestones in the lives of people you love. But at the same time, the thought of attending another baby shower as a guest, and not the guest of honor, may be more than you can bear. If this is the case, then it's perfectly fine to send your regrets along with your gift and head straight to a movie instead. You have to know and accept the limits of what you can and cannot handle gracefully and give yourself the right to opt out whenever you feel the need.

Although you may intentionally choose not to attend an abundance of child-centric events, at the same time you may begin to feel isolated. You appreciate that your friends are trying to make it easier on you, but when your entire social circle seems to revolve around children in one way or another, it doesn't leave you with a lot of other social options. No matter if you're withdrawing from your friends or gently being excluded, you feel the same—sad, lonely and desperate to be one of them. Or desperate to get away from them.

Things That Push You Over the Edge

You've taken the liberty to RSVP "no" to the child-related functions you just don't think you can make it through. It should be enough, but it isn't. There may not be actual children everywhere reminding you of your kid-free status, but there are plenty of signs and symbols cruelly pointing out that you still don't have one to call your own.

A drive through your neighborhood used to be fairly boring—maybe you'd notice if someone had recently painted their house or bought a new car. Now, all you see are those stupid giant storks seemingly everywhere as they announce a new birth around every corner. To some, they may be cute and adorable with their oversized yellow beaks carefully toting a cute blue or pink bundle, but to you they represent a static, yet disturbing, variation of Alfred Hitchcock's *The Birds*. They might not be physically attacking you, but they are pecking away, causing you pain all the same. They make you so angry you're half-tempted to mow them down with your car, and you know you'd get away with it too. Those unlucky teens in the neighborhood would surely be blamed, as they've made a sport out of smashing down everyone's mailboxes with their baseball bats.

It's not just at home where you feel the gods are laughing at your misfortune. You begin to feel like restaurants also get a kick out of taunting and teasing you. Must their menus and signage scream, "Kids Eat Free"? What sort of deal does a couple without kids get? How about a free dessert for anyone who can prove they've spent more than $25,000 trying to have a child?

Me, Myself and I

When you are trying to get pregnant, pregnant women are everywhere—at the gas station, the airport, the grocery store, the post office—everywhere. On most days, you feel happy for them and smile affectionately when they rub their "little bump." You view pregnant women as a source of inspiration—this is why you continue to struggle through fertility treatment. Someday, you'll be in line to buy stamps, and you'll be rubbing your adorable belly.

But there will also be days that you just can't bear to see another inflated belly and its blatant reminder that you are not pregnant. These are the days you'd like to drag out the wood chipper and grind all those obnoxious wooden storks into kindling. Before you place an emergency call for roadside assistance, remember this is just another bump on the fertility-treatment highway. Like driving in a bad storm, sometimes the best thing to do is pull off to the side of the road and just wait for it to pass. Before you know it, the old you will resurface, and you'll be back to your better self. The wood chipper will be replaced with a care package, complete with balloons tied to the mailbox and a perfectly wrapped gift left at her door, you secretly deliver to a new mom in the neighborhood.

Just remember, the most important person to take care of as the fertility journey drags on is you . . . whoever that may be on any given day. So on the days you feel like staying home and feeling sorry for yourself as you eat ice cream straight out of the container and watch sappy 1980s movies on TV, go ahead and get comfy. On the days you feel like throwing a baby shower for your pregnant best friend, do it. And for once in your life, worry about you first. Do whatever you can to make yourself feel good. A healthy mind, body and soul are your most valuable assets.

chapter twelve

IVF:
I Vow Not to Freak Out

Friday   Notes

- bloodwork 8 a.m. / shot 7 p.m.

Saturday   Notes   ## Sunday   Notes

- bloodwork 8 a.m. /   - bloodwork 8 a.m. /
shot 7 p.m.   shot 7 p.m.

"I think it's time you consider IVF."

These words hang in the air like the smell of bad fish. Of course, you knew it was coming. You were a trifecta flunky of the injectables/IUI program, and the sole purpose of what feels like your weekly consultation with your doctor is to discuss your next step. You knew he would say it was time to move on to IVF (in vitro fertilization), but nothing really prepared you for actually hearing the words. You never thought it would come to this.

There are no easy steps in the fertility treatment process. But making the decision to move on to the final step of a three-step process can be especially trying. You think back longingly to the days when you struggled with the decision to take Clomid or move on to injectable drugs. Child's play. Of course, those weren't easy decisions at the time, but somewhere in your subconscious, there was a degree of comfort knowing that if your attempts failed, there was always another option.

IVF is different. It's the last call for you to experience childbirth. The lights are flickering on and off, and you realize time is running out. If this doesn't work, there's nowhere else to turn—your chances of becoming a biological mother are over (or so you think).

Now you are faced with yet another fork in the road and forced to make a decision you never thought you'd have to make. You think back to the countless conversations you had over the years with friends who vehemently declared, "I would never go to such lengths as IVF to have children." At the time, you may have even agreed with them. Of course, most of these friends can stand firm with their convictions, as they were lucky enough to crank out a family of five with little effort. Remember, it's much easier to make sweeping statements about what you would and would not do when you're not actually confronted with the decision. Your opinion of IVF may suddenly change when you realize it may be the one option to get you to your ultimate goal of becoming pregnant.

While some may spend hours, day or weeks contemplating the moral and ethical implications of IVF, others may be thrilled with the opportunity it provides. For those who suffer from blocked tubes or other internal structural damage, this may be their one chance to achieve pregnancy. Other women may not find the decision to try IVF intimidating at all. In fact, they may opt to skip over step two (injectables/IUI) and move directly to IVF. This decision may be based on their ages, the higher success rates of IVF or the greater amount of control IVF provides over high-order multiples.

While injectables stimulate the ovaries to produce multiple follicles, there's no control over how many of those eggs may fertilize each cycle. On the other hand, IVF uses the same gonadotropins to stimulate the ovaries, but the eggs are removed from the body and united with sperm in a laboratory. Once the eggs have fertilized, a select number of embryos are transferred back to the uterus. By controlling the number of embryos returned to the uterus, you greatly reduce the "litter factor."

To:	Shelly <Shelly@conceptionchronicles.com>;
	Courtney <Courtney@conceptionchronicles.com>
From:	Patty <Patty@conceptionchronicles.com>
Subject:	**The Big Tomato**

Scott and I talked about it last night, and we decided we are going to try IVF. I'm a little nervous about it—the shots, the daily blood work, the intensity of it all. Even though it's a bit intimidating, I feel like we have to give it a try, so that I never have to look back and wonder "what if."

God knows, Scott and I haven't always been on the same page

throughout this ordeal, but I finally think we are completely in synch. I feel like he's the only one who really understands what this means for us.

To: Patty <Patty@conceptionchronicles.com>
From: Courtney <Courtney@conceptionchronicles.com>
CC: Shelly <Shelly@conceptionchronicles.com>
Subject: **RE: The Big Tomato**

I know this is a huge decision for you and Scott, but I completely agree that you will never have to regret not trying everything. I have a really good feeling about this.

To: Patty <Patty@conceptionchronicles.com>
From: Shelly <Shelly@conceptionchronicles.com>
CC: Courtney <Courtney@conceptionchronicles.com>
Subject: **RE: RE: The Big Tomato**

Stay positive. I think it's great you guys are moving forward. I'll be sending good thoughts your way.

The Silver Bullet

While there is no silver bullet that will guarantee your success of getting pregnant, IVF certainly has the reputation of one. We've all heard the stories: forty-five-year-old celebrity marries fifty-five-year-old husband and *boom*—twins; woman with no fallopian tubes marries husband with vasectomy and *pow*—a bouncing baby boy arrives; couple tries for eight years with no luck and *zam*—they're pregnant . . . all courtesy of a little thing called IVF.

These stories are everywhere. So much so that when you finally get over your decision to try IVF, you may be completely shocked to learn it doesn't come with a money-back guarantee. What's even more shocking are the success rates. In 1992, a law was passed requiring all U.S. clinics practicing assisted reproductive technology to report to the Centers for Disease Control detailed data on the procedures performed and the outcomes. The CDC compiles this information and publishes reports on the national averages, as well as each individual clinic's results, on their Web site at *www.cdc.gov.* Although the data may not be completely current (the government moves at a snail-like pace), the information is invaluable. Not only can you look at the national average for your age group, you can also compare the results of your clinic with others in the area to help make the best choice for your maiden IVF voyage.

As of 2005, the most current data available on the CDC Web site is from 2002. When looking at the reports, you will see they are broken down by age group and type of cycle (i.e., fresh embryos from nondonor eggs, frozen embryos from nondonor eggs and donor egg cycles). The following headlines the 2002 National Summary report from the CDC:

Type of Cycle	Age of Woman			
Fresh Nondonor Eggs or Embryos	Under 35	35–37	38–40	41–42
Number of cycles	37,591	19,110	17,454	7,733
Percentage of cycles resulting in pregnancies	43%	36%	28%	17%
Percentage of cycles resulting in live births	37%	31%	21%	11%

Shocking right? When we first started researching IVF, we expected to see success rates in the 70 to 80 percent range, not 20 to 40 percent. It's hard to look at these numbers and not feel a wave of doom and gloom, but when you consider that a "normal" couple has only a 10 to 20 percent chance of conceiving each month, it doesn't seem so terrible.

As you continue your search for an IVF clinic, you will notice some clinics do boast results that are slightly higher than average. Is it because they are a superior clinic? Maybe, maybe not. Some clinics prioritize stats over service and refuse to work with more challenging cases to ensure that their superior success rates remain intact. So use these numbers as a guideline, but don't make a decision on a clinic based strictly on their stats.

We know it's virtually impossible to think rationally about the success rates. Most likely you will immediately jump to your age-group box and think, "Oh my God, I have only a one in three chance of this working." If you find yourself approaching a birthday that will push you into the next age group, feel free to convince yourself you belong in the younger set for at least the next six months. Clearly, someone who is thirty-five and one month old has much more in common with the under thirty-five set than the thirty-five to thirty-seven group. Why should your chances of success be dragged down by the old hags in the next box?

Before you admit defeat and throw in the towel, remember these are *averages*, and your diagnosis may make your chances of success very different from others in your age group. Even though it won't be easy, try not to let yourself get too caught up in the numbers.

To put it in perspective, Babe Ruth, the Home Run King, was unquestionably one of the greatest hitters the diamond has ever seen. Yet his career batting average was .342, which means he was shuffling back to the dugout a lot more often than doing a home run victory lap after getting up to bat. In the words of The Babe, "Never let the fear of striking out get in your way." Although we're quite sure he wasn't thinking about your reproductive woes when these inspiring words passed his lips, they fit. Remember, it only takes one home run to make your dreams come true.

Cash, Check or Charge?

One of the most common misperceptions about IVF is that it is a treatment for older, rich women who put off having children earlier in life. It is often portrayed as a convenience, a choice. While that may be the case for some, it's certainly not the case for most. As you saw from the 2002 CDC statistics, there were as many women under the age of thirty-five who sought the help of IVF as there were women thirty-five to forty. And while the IVF journey would be much more manageable with a nice juicy trust fund to sink your teeth into, there are plenty of couples holding down second jobs, mortgaging their homes and borrowing money from friends and family all for a chance at IVF.

So just how much does a cycle of IVF with a 10 to 37 percent chance of success go for these days? The costs can vary widely, depending on the clinic, the prescription drugs and the necessary laboratory services. According to RESOLVE: The National Infertility Association, a typical IVF cycle may cost anywhere from $12,000 to $25,000. Looking at the success rates, it doesn't take a mathematician to figure out it may take more than one cycle before you're pregnant. Start multiplying these numbers by two or three, and we're talking a small fortune.

Show Me the Money

On your next visit to the doctor's office, you announce you are anxious to try IVF. For some reason, you expected a "you made the right decision" pep talk from the doctor, followed by his reassurances that this was going to work. Instead, he spins around in his imported leather chair and whips out a price sheet with a line-item breakdown of all the IVF costs. After briefly reviewing the costs, he tells you to set up a meeting with the clinic's financial coordinator to verify how you plan to pay. Only after you are a documented paying customer will you be permitted to sign up for the prerequisite IVF class.

It's a sad reality, but the fertility medical community is a business. Yes, they are there to help you have a baby, but they are also there to make enough money for sporty little convertibles with license plates that cleverly work in the initials "MD." Some clinics go so far as to post warnings in every exam room that your cycle will be canceled if it turns out your insurance company needed to preapprove your treatment. Who cares if you have twenty eggs about ready to burst out of your ovaries? No money, no treatment.

If you're lucky, you will have some level of insurance coverage for IVF. Even if your insurance has covered all of your treatment up until this point, you must carefully review the policy, because it is not uncommon for IVF to be excluded. Some plans only cover a portion of the treatment, such as the procedure, the monitoring or the drugs, and you are responsible for the balance. Your portion of the costs can add up quickly, so make sure you know exactly what you're getting into before you sign on the bottom line. If you're without insurance or your clinic does not accept your plan, you may be expected to pay in full before any treatment begins.

Advocacy groups have been lobbying for years for legislation requiring insurance companies to provide fertility treatment coverage. As of right now, there are no federal laws in place, but several states have passed legislation that mandates some level of fertility treatment coverage. If your current plan doesn't include IVF, check with *www.resolve.org* or your local state government to see if your state is one that requires coverage.

If you exhaust all insurance options and come up empty, there are still some alternatives to help ease the burden. Some clinics may accept donations of unused medications from patients who have completed their treatment and offer them to self-pay patients for free to help offset some of the expense. Clinics should also be able to put you in touch with discount mail-order pharmacies, which should help defray a portion of the shocking drug costs.

Some clinics even offer a "shared egg" program, where a woman uses half of her eggs retrieved and donates the other half for discounted treatment. This can be a good financial option for both the donor and the recipient, but it can also create a whole new set of issues.

In many industries, there are often significant price discounts given to companies for large purchases of goods or services. The medical community is no different. One of the greatest injustices in medicine today is the insurance industry's price break. If a doctor agrees to work with an insurance provider, he commits to the fee schedule the insurance company provides. While you may be charged $250 as a self-pay patient for an ultrasound, the insurance company may only agree to a $75 rate, and that's what they pay . . . period.

So the multimillion-dollar insurance company gets the price break, while you, the "hard working, we'll put off getting a new car another few years so we can afford this" patient, make up the difference on the P&L by paying top dollar. This makes absolutely no sense, but it's happening. Proving there are still some caring doctors left in the world, some clinics will offer their self-pay patients a discount, and in some cases, they may even agree to accept the rock-bottom insurance rates. While you may feel a bit uncomfortable negotiating the cost of a vaginal ultrasound, believe us, you won't be the first to do so. It certainly can't hurt to ask. The answer may be "no," but then again, it may also be a big-fat-thousand-dollars-in-your-pocket "yes."

Ready, Set, Wait

After trudging through a sea of research material, selecting a clinic and proving your ability to pay cold, hard cash for services, you are anxious to get going. You stop by the receptionist's desk, and after patiently waiting while she explains how she got her lemon meringue pie so light and fluffy to the rest of the loitering staff, you finally blurt out you need an appointment to discuss your medications for IVF. She pulls out the calendar and tells you she can squeeze you in a week from Tuesday, but there are a few things you need to do before you can start your cycle. Then she hands you an information packet that puts the introductory information to shame. The "Where Dreams Come True" folder should be more appropriately labeled "Where Dreams Come True *IF* You Hand Over Your Wallet." The double-sided IVF packet is crammed on one side with information, consents and instructions. The opposite pocket may as well have a big dollar sign embossed on it, because this side is reserved for even more detailed information about how much all of this is going to cost, along with forms that basically say they will sell you into slavery if you don't pay. Aren't you supposed to be making a new life, not signing your own away?

Buried deep in the packet is a checklist of things that must be done before you can begin IVF. This is where the fun begins and your free time ends. There are tests that must be done on certain days of your cycle, classes that are offered conveniently only one day a week in the middle of the day and procedures that must be scheduled days apart from other tests. All in all, it's a scheduling nightmare, so if you're working, this is probably the time to fess up to your boss, because the odds of your getting to work on a timely basis for the foreseeable future are slim. Your husband, on the other hand, will simply have to drop off another semen sample and have a blood test at his convenience. Oh well, at least he has to do something.

Back to School

Soon you find yourself back in the staff cafeteria, only this time it's for IVF class. Unlike the awkward silence of the injections class, this group seems overly chatty and a little too eager to share their personal medical histories. This class will most likely be your first glimpse into the secret society of IVF. While you may be the type of person who gets in and out of doctor's appointments without making eye contact, never mind small talk, with anyone in the lobby, don't be surprised if you are exchanging numbers with the low sperm motility couple by the end of class. It's a strange phenomenon; there's an instant bond between those who have been through hell and arrived at the same place: IVF.

When class gets underway, you learn there are six phases to IVF: suppression, stimulation, egg retrieval, fertilization, embryo transfer and follow-up blood work. The nurse explains you will come into the office for baseline blood work and an ultrasound when you get your period. If all looks good, the doctor will put you on birth control pills. What?! You've got to be kidding me. You've spent the last months, maybe years, trying to get pregnant, and now you're expected to take the pill? Relax. It's only temporary. The doctor basically needs to shut down your natural cycle so he can take over. Think of it as remote control.

As you start wondering how many days it will take to suppress your system, the nurse continues and announces the suppression phase can take anywhere from two to six weeks. This is the first of many facts that will make your ears perk up. Two to six weeks? Crap. If you're suppressed for six weeks, it's definitely going to cut into your spring ski vacation that's already paid in full. When you ask the nurse if you have any say in the amount of time you are suppressed, she flatly says, "No. If you can't commit to the schedule, you should cancel and try again next month." Note to self:

Don't make any plans until the next century or until bouncing baby arrives.

Some clinics actually do all of their IVF procedures at one time. They only take a limited amount of patients for each cycle, so women must commit in advance to predetermined dates. Usually it's the larger, highly sought-after clinics that schedule this way. Patients may find themselves signing up for the first available IVF cycle, which may be six months down the road. Once their number is finally called, the women are put on birth control pills until their cycles are synchronized with the rest of the patients in the group. Wouldn't Henry Ford be proud to know the assembly line is not just for cars anymore?

Class continues, and the nurse explains that once your body is suppressed, you'll move on to the stimulation phase. If you've already done injectables/IUI, this is old news. You know the drill—gonadotropins are used to stimulate the ovaries to produce multiple follicles. The main difference with IVF is doctors can be much more aggressive with the medication because the eggs will be removed from the body. But there is still the risk of hyperstimulation, so constant monitoring is crucial.

This brings us to the point everyone is anxiously awaiting. The nurse rolls down the familiar poster of the female anatomy and begins to explain exactly how your eggs will be leaving your body. In a matter-of-fact tone, she begins, "A long needle is inserted into the vagina, along with an ultrasound probe to guide the way. The needle is poked through the back wall of the vagina, into the ovary and pierces each individual follicle. Then, the fluid that contains the egg is extracted from each follicle. Any questions?"

"Are you conscious during the retrieval?" some brave soul asks on behalf of every woman in the room. Much to the relief of the nail-biting crowd, the nurse tells you this procedure is done under general anesthesia.

After the buzz settles down in the room about how scary egg retrieval is, the nurse continues. "Once the eggs are retrieved, they are shown to their new home, complete with 360-degree views ... the petri dish. They will be joined shortly thereafter by your husband's sperm. Hopefully, they will hit it off and unite, creating a fertilized embryo. Three to five days later, the embryos will be transferred back to your warm, comfy uterus. The embryo transfer is very similar to artificial insemination; it's a relatively simple procedure. You will be awake as a catheter is guided through your cervix and into your uterus, where your embryos will be left to snuggle in for the next nine months."

"And that's it," the nurse cheerfully proclaims. "After the transfer, you will return four days later to check your blood levels and the week after that for the pregnancy test. It's not so bad, right?" she asks. Aside from the daily trips to the doctor's office, the endless shots at home, the minor surgery and the intrusive procedure to get everything back to where it never should have left in the first place, you guess she's right. Maybe it won't be so bad. As you leave the class, the nurse tells you to be sure to stop by the receptionist to schedule an appointment to get your drug protocol.

IVF Spring Training

The time between making the decision to do IVF and actually starting IVF can feel like an eternity. You're already mentally committed to getting started, so treading water as you endure test after test can be excruciating. Rather than agonizing day after day, try to use this time productively to get yourself in the best mental and physical health for the cycle. If you haven't already, now's definitely the time to be good to yourself. Cut back on drive-through dinners, and treat yourself to a new cookbook that features delicious recipes packed with fresh seasonal fruits and vegetables. Take a nice long walk every day or sign up for a mind/body stress-management class. Even if you aren't feeling the stress right now, you will, so why not be prepared with techniques to calm your mind and body.

One of the most important things you can do is find a certified acupuncturist. While your doctor may or may not be a big believer in acupuncture, there have been studies that show acupuncture can help with fertility treatment by increasing blood flow to the uterus and stimulating fertility hormones. Some leading doctors in the field have called for more detailed research around the fertility-boosting effects of acupuncture because they've seen promising results in their own practices, but there has yet to be a definitive clinical study.

As for acupuncture, we don't need a room full of pocket-protecting Ph.D.s to convince us. One of our TTCs, who was only thirty years old at the time, was horrified after her first IVF cycle when she was told she had the eggs of a forty-five-year-old woman. She tried two more cycles of IVF, which were both unsuccessful. Her doctor told her there was very little hope for her, given the quality of her eggs. Unwilling to give up, she decided to take a break from the craziness and try something a little less mainstream. She found an acupuncturist and went religiously for the next few months. After feeling rejuvenated, she decided to give IVF one last shot. There wasn't a drastic change, but things went a little more smoothly. She responded to the medication a little bit better, she had a few more eggs and she ended up with two good embryos. Were they perfect? No. Did they result in the perfect family she always wanted? Yes. She gave birth to healthy twins, a boy and a girl.

Even if there isn't a three-hundred page research paper in the bowels of the medical library touting the benefits of acupuncture, what do you have to lose? Ask your doctor for a recommendation, and get started right away. The effects of acupuncture are cumulative, so don't run in two days before your egg retrieval and expect a miracle. But if you make the effort and attend appointments regularly, it may just give your body the extra boost it needs for success.

To:	Shelly <Shelly@conceptionchronicles.com>;
	Courtney <Courtney@conceptionchronicles.com>
From:	Patty <Patty@conceptionchronicles.com>
Subject:	**I'm cured!**

I've officially overcome my needle phobia . . . I'm seeing an acupuncturist! For someone who couldn't look at a needle w/out getting faint, I am now willingly paying someone to stick more pins in me than a voodoo doll. The sick thing is, I really like it.

To:	Patty <Patty@conceptionchronicles.com>
From:	Shelly <Shelly@conceptionchronicles.com>
Cc:	Courtney <Courtney@conceptionchronicles.com>
Subject:	**RE: I'm cured!**

Now that you've overcome your fear, does this mean we'll be seeing a shamrock tattoo on your butt?

Honey, It's Time

Finally! It's time. The day you've been waiting for has finally arrived. You have an appointment with your doctor to review your protocol and sign the necessary waivers for IVF. You've read through the stack of consent forms countless times, contemplating the implications of each one. You gave them to your husband last week to review and reminded him on his way out the door this morning to make sure he brings them to the appointment. The waivers require witnesses, and if they are not signed in the doctor's presence, they will have to be notarized to verify the signatures. You don't want anything to slow down the process. You want this done and off your list when you walk out of the office this afternoon.

At your appointment, the doctor walks you through your protocol. The protocol basically lays out exactly what drugs you'll be taking and when you'll be taking them. You're a little surprised to see you'll be getting injections twice a day, morning and evening. What's even more disturbing is that some of the drugs can't be mixed, so you may have to take two or three shots at a time. Aside from the frequency of shots, nothing else really comes as a big surprise. You've been spending more and more time on the fertility bulletin boards, so you had a pretty good idea of what to expect. You can't wait to get home and post your protocol to see if anyone else did the same thing, and if they did, was it successful?

After discussing your protocol, the doctor asks if you read the consent forms and if you brought them with you to sign. After fumbling in his briefcase for what feels like an eternity, your husband proudly holds up the slightly crumbled forms. The doctor reads through the basics of each one before asking you to sign. The first one is your consent to use the medication. Yes, you know there are risks associated with hyperstimulation, but you are accepting the risks and agree to take the medication. You both sign.

The next consent is specifically geared toward the IVF procedure. By signing this form, you are basically giving your consent to do IVF. Yes, you agree to have your eggs removed; yes, you agree to have them fertilized with your husband's sperm; and yes, you agree to have them placed back into your uterus. We're not exactly sure how someone could sneak an embryo into your uterus, but just in case, the bases are covered. In addition, you have the choice to accept or deny such procedures as assisted egg hatching and embryo freezing. By clearly establishing your preferences up front, you will not be confronted with these decisions in the middle of your treatment.

The last form is the custody form. If you don't actually have children, odds are you haven't spent a lot of time sitting around contemplating custody. That is, until today. When the doctor pulls out the last form and asks who gets custody of the frozen embryos if you happen to get divorced, your husband replies, "Hmmm, I never really thought of that." You bark back, "You never really thought of it because you never bothered to read the forms." After an awkward silence, your doctor jots a note in the file and asks for your decision. Then it's on to the even cheerier subject of who gets your snow babies if you both die. You've always known who would get your grandmother's china, your favorite heirlooms and your killer CD collection, but who has the perfect uterus for your unborn children?

Finally, the last question. What if one of you dies? Does the surviving spouse get the embryos or should they be destroyed? You're a little surprised when your husband dismissively says, "What would I do with them?" When you tell him he can implant them in his new twenty-five-year-old wife so you can live on forever, the doctor makes another note in the file. What the hell is he writing? Doesn't he realize you've been making inappropriate jokes your entire life as a way to break tension? You sit up a little straighter, and in your most grown-up voice, you agree with your husband on the decision and sign on the dotted line.

You're done. Your doctor hands over the stack of prescriptions for your drugs and tells you to meet with the nurse to make sure it is all ordered correctly. Make sure to keep a copy of all the prescriptions for your files and to verify that what you receive from the pharmacy is correct. You start birth control pills in the morning.

Suppression

Well, here it goes. You swallow the first birth control pill. To add insult to injury, your insurance doesn't cover birth control, so last night you had to shell out fifty bucks for something that would prevent you from getting pregnant. Oh, the irony.

Sex on demand is history. You're now at a place where sex will not even factor into your conception efforts. On the one hand, you're relieved; you've blown through more candles than you care to remember and still have nothing to show for them. On the other hand, you're slightly disappointed. Call yourself an optimist, but you've been secretly hoping for a miracle every step of the way. You've heard countless stories of women who were told they'd never get pregnant without IVF, yet somehow they end up conceiving while they're waiting for their treatment to start. Unfortunately, you weren't one of them, so it's time to focus on your reality and pop another pill.

Even when doing artificial insemination, most of us were busy working on a Plan B. What if I ovulated early? What if I ovulated late? What if the sperm count wasn't good on the day of insemination? Not to worry. All bases were covered with Plan B. The Aggressive Ovulator continued to maintain a rigid sex-on-demand schedule in addition to IUI and managed all at-home activities accordingly. But now, sex has absolutely no role in achieving pregnancy with IVF. Some women actually feel a sense of relief when they start taking birth control pills. For once, destiny is completely out of their hands. You may feel so happy that there is no underlying motivation for your bedroom activities that you resume the "pre trying to get pregnant" you and swing from the chandelier. Or you may have a slightly more negative reaction and think, "Why bother? I can't get pregnant anyway," and freeze up like a Frigidaire. However you're feeling, go with it. This is no time to be worrying about what's right or wrong. Do what feels right to you.

Special Delivery

One day the FedEx truck pulls up to your door, and you immediately think, "Hurray, my new J. Crew flip-flops are here." As you open the door to meet the driver, all you can see is a large box and a clipboard dangling from a hairy arm. As the clipboard is extended with the flick of a wrist, a muffled voice says, "Please sign on line five." You scribble your name and drag the box inside. It's not until you study the return address label that you realize what the package is. It's your fertility drugs from the discount pharmacy.

When you went through your protocol, you knew you'd be taking several different drugs, but nothing prepared you for the vision of needles, syringes, medications and supplies that burst out of the box the minute you broke the seal. Long needles, short needles, skinny needles, fat needles . . . all mixed together among cotton balls, alcohol swabs, and boxes and boxes of drugs. The reality is starting to set in: this is really happening.

The first thing you must do is verify everything that was sent to you against the prescriptions. Once you've done that, read the storage directions for each medication. Some drugs need to be stored in the refrigerator, while others need to be kept at room temperature. To make your life a little easier, you may want to run out and get some type of organizer. A plastic storage bin with multiple compartments or a jewelry organizer with several drawers will do the trick. Then you can start rummaging through the piles of needles, sort them by medication and store them separately in labeled drawers. This all may sound a bit anal, but if you're doing a shot first thing in the morning, the last thing you want to do is accidentally stick yourself with a needle the size of a screwdriver that was only meant to extract medication, not inject.

Now it's time to make room in the fridge. The shelf that was once reserved for soda and beer is plowed clear to make room for your pallet of drugs. If you have people who come in and out of your house and who don't think twice about rummaging around for food and beverages, plan accordingly. Maybe you can cleverly disguise your medicinal goodies in Tupperware labeled, "brussels sprouts." That ought to keep the crowd away.

Depending on your protocol, you may actually begin your injections during this phase. Your doctor may have you on a medication, like Lupron, to help further suppress your system. At this point, you couldn't care less if the medication is a shot, a pill or a suppository; you just want to get going.

Stimulation

Okay, you take that back. You'd trade your left arm (or at least your husband's left arm) for a chewable gonadotropin. Now that you've moved on to the stimulation phase, you're taking multiple shots both morning and night. Add that to the fact that you're running to the doctor's office every day for blood work, which also requires multiple stabs because your veins retract like a startled tortoise the minute the nurse walks in the room, and you've had just about enough of the poking.

The daily ultrasounds are a different story. The probe has barely touched your skin when you start firing questions at the technician. Is that a follicle? How big is it? How big should it be? How many are there? How many should there be?

Most ultrasound technicians have the finely honed communication skills of a seasoned politician. While they will happily answer the facts—how many follicles you have and how big they are—speculative questions slide right off of them as if they were made of Teflon. As much as you ask, they are not going to tell you whether you are an over- or underachiever in egg production. They will leave that up to the doctor.

Even though the ultrasound technicians won't weigh in on your daily progress, there are plenty of others who will. First, there is your new circle of friends, the IVF sisterhood. Most clinics designate a certain time, usually very early in the morning, that is strictly reserved for IVF patients' daily blood work and ultrasound. This helps ease the time commitment—IVF patients are in and out before the crazy day of regular patients begins. Aside from scheduling, the added benefit is the creation of an IVF sisterhood. On the first few days, you may tiptoe in and head straight to the magazine rack, but after seeing the same women in the lobby day after day, you're bound to strike up a conversation and maybe even a friendship.

You'll be amazed at how quickly you feel comfortable sharing your personal struggle with someone who was a complete stranger only days before. The women who are a few days, or even a few weeks, ahead of you in their treatment can provide a sneak preview of what's to come. Just hearing firsthand that egg retrieval wasn't nearly as bad as expected from someone who actually had her eggs retrieved can be a huge relief.

One of our TTCs was going through her first cycle of IVF and immediately bonded with her IVF waiting-room sisters. The group looked forward to reporting and hearing each other's progress each morning. One day, one of the women announced she had a funny lump where she had injected her medication the night before. Next thing you know, she dropped her drawers right in the waiting room for a little show and tell. When the nurse came out to call the next patient, she found four women struggling for a diagnosis as they huddled around a woman in powder blue satin panties. Clearly, the nurse had seen it all, as she didn't even flinch but simply said, "Grab your pants, and let's get someone with a medical degree to take a look."

The Dailies

Throughout the stimulation phase, you will typically get your medication instructions on a day-to-day basis. After the doctor reviews the results of your daily tests, he will adjust the medication accordingly and have someone from the office call you with your dosage for the evening and the next morning. Then it's back to the office the next morning to do it all over again.

The amount of time it takes to be stimulated varies widely based on the individual and the protocol, but it typically ranges from eight to sixteen days. Regardless of how many days you are taking the stimulants, the daily trips to the office are brutal. One day you go in and everything seems to be going according to schedule. Hurray! You're convinced this is going to work. The next day you go in and things are disastrous: you don't have enough follicles, they aren't growing and so forth. Now you're convinced your cycle is going to be canceled. These are the days you may not want to report your performance to the team waiting in the lobby. You'll feel even worse when you hear that someone who started her cycle three days after you is further along with her stimulation.

Time for the bulletin boards. You may find carpal tunnel syndrome setting in as you sit again frantically posting your most recent results on the board. When you first started posting, you struggled with all the acronyms, but now they fly off your fingers like pig Latin used to fly off your lips in eighth grade. It's a new language, and you're fluent. You've even taken the liberty to add a little more flavor to the cyberlingo with a few acronyms of your own:

TS	This Sucks
SF	Stinkin' Follicles
SA	Sore Ass
LOE	Lazy Old Eggs
WM	Why Me?

Just when you decide to write off the cycle as a failure, you go in to find your sluggish follicles have woken up and caught up with the rest of the world. Things are looking good again.

You should expect to have at least three moments of sheer terror throughout the stimulation process. If you're prepared, it may not be as shocking when you hear the words, "Hmmm, we really expected you to react more quickly to the medication." Remember, you're under constant monitoring for a reason. If you don't react as expected, your medication will be adjusted each day to get you where you need to go. And it only takes one egg to make a beautiful baby.

Egg Retrieval

Ding. You're done.

You're serving up more eggs than the Lakeside Diner, and it's time to get them out. This is the moment you've been waiting for. When the nurse calls with your daily instructions, she tells you to stop taking your stimulants. Then she tells you what time you are scheduled for your retrieval and exactly what time you must take your hCG trigger shot. While it may sound crazy to wake up at 3:05 A.M. for a shot, you must do *exactly* what she says. The hCG is timed around the retrieval, taking it too early or too late can ruin the whole cycle.

You will be told not to eat or drink anything after midnight the evening before the retrieval, because you will be put under anesthesia. One of our TTCs was telling her husband how thirsty and hungry she was as they drove to their appointment. "Maybe we'll stop at the diner on the way home," her husband said. Not wanting to start a fight on one of the most important days of their life, she did her best to hold back the "you're an idiot" tone in her voice when she replied, "I'm not sure after being put under general anesthesia, having ten holes poked in my vagina and having all my eggs sucked out I'll be up for a greasy western omelet with fries." Clearly, she didn't try hard enough, because her husband snapped back, "Well, I don't know. I've never been through IVH before either." No, this is not a typo the editor sloppily overlooked. Yes, he called IVF, IVH. Chalking it up to the pure fear of what lay ahead, they actually laughed for the first time that day.

Who Are You?

One of the most unsettling things about the egg-retrieval procedure is it may not be done by your doctor. There are a million reasons why this may happen, none of which will comfort you. Just remind yourself over and over that you trust your doctor, and he is having the most qualified person do the procedure.

After meeting the staff who will perform the procedure, an IV is started, and you are given a medication that makes you feel like you've had one too many martinis. Once you are comfortably settled onto the procedure table, someone from the embryology lab comes in and asks you to verify your name and social security number (this is to avoid any chance of your eggs cheating on your husband's sperm). As you start drunkenly babbling on about how much better you feel knowing there's a system in place so they don't mix up your eggs with someone else's, the anesthesiologist squeezes another tube of liquid into your IV and you're out.

While you're in dreamland, your husband is watching *Pornville*. It's time for him to produce his sample. We can't imagine the pressure our poor husbands feel. Not only is this the first time he has to "perform" outside the home, it's also a sterile environment, so he has to wear paper booties over his shoes. Couple that with the fact that the last image he has of you is you stumbling to the operating room wearing a hairnet and a rumpled paper gown. The poor guy has his work cut out for him. Thus, we say that he deserves a little porn. For God's sake, give him a line of dancing, naked girls if that's what it takes.

Most clinics understand the pressure husbands feel, and they do their best to accommodate. But just like your mother can never pick out a sweater you'd ever wear in public, so too do the clinics fall a bit short with their efforts. Maybe it's the fact that your husband knows the magazines have been pawed over by countless other masturbators or the video selection is circa 1980, but the props provided may not do it for him. Hopefully he has a strong imagination. Worst-case scenario, the doctors can extract the semen from him with a needle. Just hearing those words usually does the trick. Somehow your husband manages to pull through in the clutch.

Can You Open Your Eyes?

The next thing you know, you are back in recovery. In the distance, you hear someone asking you to open your eyes, but you have more pressing issues on your mind. Before you show any sign of life, you shock the recovery team by shouting out, "How many eggs did you retrieve?" Even if they tell you, you won't remember, so make sure your husband is briefed on his responsibility to corner the doctor after the retrieval to get all the details.

After a few sips of water and some random chitchatting with the nurses, you are free to go. You'll be given written instructions and told to take it easy for the next few days. You'll also be reminded to start your progesterone shots that night.

The Holy-Shit Shot

The moment you've been dreading since first laying eyes on the one-and-a-half-inch needle at injections class is here. If you had good news at the retrieval, you may feel a sense of euphoria that may make you believe the shot won't be too bad. It will.

There's no way to sugarcoat it—the intramuscular needles suck. The only thing you can do is lessen the impact of the suckiness.

Your husband is going to be a nervous wreck, and odds are it's going to take some time before he masters the technique. The bad news is, it's your behind that will be suffering through the mishaps during the early amateur days.

Break out your written instructions from class and follow them step-by-step. To lessen the pain, ice the area for a good five minutes before you give your husband the thumbs-up to proceed. Try deep breathing and counting with each inhale and exhale to calm your mind. Once it's over, massage the area (or better yet have your husband massage the area) with a warm cloth, or sit on a heating pad. Because progesterone comes in an oil base, it has a tendency to form nodules if it is not warmed and worked into the muscle.

Typically, progestrone is prescribed with a sesame oil base, but it is also available in other oils, such as cottonseed, if you have an allergic reaction. So don't think you're off the hook if you break out in hives like one of our TTCs did shortly after starting her Holy Shit shots. Her doctor simply switched the prescription to a new oil base, and she was right back on schedule.

We're not going to say the Holy Shit shot ever gets easy, but it does get better. Take it one day at a time, and you'll get through it.

Fertilization

The day after your retrieval, you will receive a call telling you how many eggs were mature and how many fertilized. You and your husband will spend every minute up until that call playing out different scenarios: What if none fertilize? What if they all fertilize? What if the eggs are bad? What if the sperm is bad? Your entire house could burn down around you, and you would not leave your post next to the phone. Your heart pounds every time it rings, only to be disappointed by the phone company offering a new long-distance rate.

Finally, you get the news. The lab calls to tell you how many embryos you have. Unfortunately, at this point, that's all they can tell you. It's too early to tell if they're good or bad, you just know they made it this far. The lab may call you back in a few days to rate the embryos, or you may get the information when you go in for your transfer. Whether the news is better or worse than you expected, you are excited your egg and your husband's sperm have united to create a life. At least you made it this far. It gives you hope that things may just work out after all.

Embryo Transfer

Three to five days later, you will be instructed to come back to the clinic for your embryo transfer. Although a three-day transfer is standard, some clinics wait until day five when the embryo reaches the *blastocyst stage*, or the point when the embryo begins to hatch out of its shell.

The advantages and disadvantages of the day-three versus the day-five transfer are a source of debate within the medical community. Proponents of the blastocyst transfer claim the longer waiting period weeds out the weaker embryos, and only the strongest, most viable embryos remain. These doctors tout the higher success rates of the blastocyst transfer and the reduced risks of high-order multiples because fewer embryos are transferred back to the uterus on a day-five transfer.

Other doctors argue that many viable embryos, which could have survived if transferred to the uterus earlier, are lost between days three and five in the lab. They claim an embryo is more likely to thrive in its natural environment rather than in a lab and should be returned to the uterus as soon as possible.

Some labs will only consider doing a blastocyst transfer if you have a large number of good-quality embryos. Many labs don't have the expertise to develop the embryo to day five, as it is a very delicate and complicated procedure. While the higher success rates and the need to transfer fewer blastocyst embryos may sound appealing, talk to your doctor about your personal circumstances before making any decisions. If you opt to wait for a five-day transfer, you run the risk of losing all the embryos along the way. Your doctor should be able to tell you if you are a candidate for a blastocyst transfer based on the number and quality of embryos you produce.

We'll Be with You in a Minute

"How many are you going to transfer?" is the question of the day. Hopefully, you had multiple eggs fertilize, so there's a decision to be made. There's nothing worse than waiting to hear if your little guys survived the last two days. As you wait for the doctor and embryologist to come in with the report, you brace yourself for the worst possible news.

"They wouldn't make me get naked and wait in this room for half an hour if they were only going to tell me none of them made it, would they? It must mean we have at least one. Please, let there be one. It only takes one." You break down every possible scenario with your husband and decide how many embryos you will transfer under each situation. All of this speculation is basically useless until you have the facts, but at least it keeps your husband seated in a chair rather than snooping around in the speculum drawer.

Finally, the embryologist comes in and tells you how many embryos you have and how they are graded. Don't be surprised if you were told you had four eggs fertilize only to learn you now have five embryos. Sometimes an egg may not be quite mature enough to fertilize at the time of retrieval, but it continues to mature and subsequently fertilizes the next day. And don't be discouraged if you expected to have four eggs and find out on the day of your retrieval you "only" have two. Remember, it only takes one.

Most, but not all, clinics grade embryo quality based on the number of cells and the amount of fragmentation. When the sperm joins with the egg, the cell splits into two cells. As the cells continue to grow and divide, sometimes tiny pieces break off creating fragmentation. By a day-three transfer, an embryo is typically anywhere from four to eight cells. The embryologist grades the embryos based on the number of cells, the consistency of the cell sizes, the roundness of the cells and the level of fragmentation.

Don't panic if your embryos are average students. Every doctor will tell you stories of patients who had less-than-perfect embryos that resulted in beyond-perfect babies. Unfortunately, the reverse side is true too: even if you have an A+ embryo, you are not guaranteed success. The rating system has a tendency to give a false sense of security (or insecurity). The best thing to do is talk to your doctor and the embryologist about your personal situation before you make a decision about how many embryos to transfer. After that, don't look back and second-guess your decision for the next two weeks. Be confident that you did the right thing.

Table for Two or Three or Four?

Once everyone agrees on how many embryos to transfer, you will be asked to sign yet another form confirming your decision. Then it's time for the transfer. The actual procedure is very similar to an IUI. The only real difference is you are required to have a full bladder for the transfer. Once the bladder is inflated, it pushes on the cervix, which makes inserting the catheter much easier.

Most clinics will not give you a specific amount of water to drink, because every woman's bladder has a different capacity, but they will tell you to be "uncomfortably full." One of our TTCs was so concerned she hadn't drunk enough, she just kept guzzling water right up until the moment the doctor walked into the room. When the nurse put the ultrasound paddle on her stomach, she said, "Wow, you must really have to go to the bathroom." Of course, she had to go to the bathroom; wasn't that the point?

Our advice is to pace yourself. You shouldn't be writhing in pain as you try to suppress the urge to pee all over the table, but a thimble of water's not going to do the trick either. Start drinking about a half hour before your appointment. If you're not full enough when it's time for the procedure, you'll be handed a bottle of water and told to slug it back.

Follow-Up Blood Work

Before you know it, the procedure is over, and you are sent home to agonize for the next two weeks. Everything is a sign. A bird nests outside your office window, and you see two squawking heads peep out—you're having twins. One of your cycle buddies on the bulletin board, who had the same exact protocol you did, posts a BFN (Big Fat Negative)—you're not pregnant. Two more of your friends announce they're pregnant; good things come in threes—you're definitely next.

Stop. Allow yourself to breathe. Take heart in the fact you've made it this far. In two weeks, you'll have your answer. Try to remain positive. You know there are no guarantees, but for every futile attempt at conception, there are stories of new life. You will never have to ask yourself the "what if?" question years from now when it truly is too late. You took a chance, and you did everything you could.

This is not the last step in your journey to motherhood. You are wiser now than when you began your quest. Although you would be devastated if this cycle of IVF didn't work, it's not the end of the road. There are still plenty of options.

To:	Courtney <Courtney@conceptionchronicles.com>; Shelly <Shelly@conceptionchronicles.com>
From:	Patty <Patty@conceptionchronicles.com>
Subject:	**Keep your fingers crossed**

Well, we made it through IVF. It took me a while to get here, and I really, really want this to work, but if it doesn't, I know I'm going to be okay. I finally feel like I've come to a good place with this whole process. We've done everything we possibly can, and now it's out of our hands.

To:	Patty <Patty@conceptionchronicles.com>
From:	Shelly <Shelly@conceptionchronicles.com>
Cc:	Courtney <Courtney@conceptionchronicles.com>
Subject:	**RE: Keep your fingers crossed**

You made it. I'm sure everything is going to work out—you have the right attitude. I'll keep sending good vibes your way. Keep us posted.

To:	Patty <Patty@conceptionchronicles.com>
From:	Courtney <Courtney@conceptionchronicles.com>
cc:	Shelly <Shelly@conceptionchronicles.com>
Subject:	**RE: RE: Keep your fingers crossed**

I know it's been a rough road, but you've made it this far. Hang in there.

chapter thirteen

There's More Than One Road to Motherhood

Monday	Notes

- 8 p.m. Meet Lisa & Todd at airport to welcome their new baby.

- 8:30 p.m. Flight 810 arrives from China.

Tuesday	Notes	Wednesday	Notes

If It Takes a Village to Raise a Child, How Many Does It Take to Make One?

At some point, you may find yourself staring eye to eye with fertility treatment failure, even after enduring the most aggressive procedures. When you think back to your feelings before starting IVF, you thought of it as a last resort, an extreme option, but you certainly never thought it would fail . . . over and over again. But now here you are, at least you think it's you, trying to process the words you heard earlier in the doctor's office: "Traditional fertility treatment is no longer an option for you. There's no point continuing down this path. You may want to consider adoption or third-party reproductive assistance."

WHAT?!!!!!!!!!!!

Third-party reproductive assistance? You thought the doctors, nurses, phlebotomists and embryologists were the third party. It was hard enough to move your baby-making efforts from the two-party bedroom festivities to the third-, fourth- and fifth-party efforts of the cold, sterile fertility clinic. Who's left?

Before you can even begin to consider the alternatives, you must first take some time to digest your situation and grieve the loss of having a traditional biological child. For years, you've dreamed of having a baby. You wondered if your child would have your hazel eyes and your husband's dimples. Would your baby be blessed with his sense of humor or saddled with your stubbornness? You've spent hours imagining your blended features and personalities and couldn't wait to see who and what your child would become.

Now you're faced with the most devastating situation imaginable and will most likely struggle with the options and how they'll define your future path. It may be a good time to take a few months off and understand that, although you have failed in your attempts up until this point, your course may just need to be altered. Your dream to have a child may not be what it was, but under different circumstances, it can still come true.

Top-Security Clearance Required

And you thought people had something to say about assisted reproductive technology (ART)? You ain't seen nothing yet. If you're at a dinner party that's as bland as the bread, just toss out the concept of "egg donor" or "surrogate mother" and see what happens. There's one thing for certain, people are sure to have an opinion. It's going to be extreme and, most likely, misinformed. Not once have we heard someone say, "Hmmm, congratulations," after hearing you are carrying a baby who began as a donated frozen embryo. They're more likely thinking, "How dare you play God?"

You can't really blame them. People tend to be uncomfortable with things they don't fully understand. Third-party reproduction has not been around very long and is far from gaining mainstream acceptance. It may bode well in Hollywood, California, but they may not be ready for it in Hollywood, Maryland. The mother of one of our TTCs was thrilled at the prospect of becoming a first-time grandmother. As every other mother does, she bragged to all of her friends that her daughter was expecting, with twins no less. There was just one tiny detail she left out when gabbing with her coffee klatch—another woman was carrying the babies.

Be forewarned. The world at large, and more important, your world, may not be ready to embrace the measures you are prepared to take to have a child. No one who desperately wants a child should be denied the right of motherhood, and it's not for others to judge the decisions you make as to how you may get there. Unfortunately, the rest of the world doesn't always agree. No one can ever know or understand your life and what you think in your heart is right for you. No doubt the decisions you make will cause you stress along the way, but try not to second-guess yourself knowing the choices you are making are based in love. The best advice is to proceed with caution. It may be best to make the most intimate information available on a need-to-know basis.

Party of the First Part

While it's easy to get caught up in the excitement of another door opening toward motherhood, you can't let your emotions get the best of you. You must keep a level head and remain focused on the monotonous legal process that accompanies these opportunities.

Laws for adoption and third-party reproduction vary widely from state to state. Contracts, consent periods and parental rights are just a few of the critical issues that must be addressed by you, along with an experienced attorney who specializes in these disciplines. It's your responsibility to take ownership of the process and understand the surrounding issues. Thorough research will not only make you better informed, it will also help you make better decisions.

It May Not Be Golden, but It's an Egg: Egg Donation

When your doctor tells you there is little chance of conception using your own eggs, you may wonder how you will go on. If you've been told your ovarian reserve is diminished, you're perimenopausal or you have problems with ovarian function, then a donor egg may be your best chance at conceiving. In a million years, you never thought you'd be faced with the decision to use an egg donor. You don't know anyone who donates blood these days, let alone an egg. Sure, you've had friends who've done IVF, but you always assumed the eggs were home grown.

This may come as a bit of a surprise, but egg donation is happening a lot more than you may know. The 1997 American Society of Reproductive Medicine and Society of Assisted Reproductive Technology (ASRM/SART) registry reported that approximately one out of every ten ART cycles used donor eggs.

Couples may struggle with the decision to use donor eggs, but in the end they may decide it is their best option. A woman's hesitation about the lack of her genetic bond is often balanced with her eagerness to experience pregnancy and childbirth. While it's not ideal, couples may take solace knowing there is a biological connection to their child through the genetic link with the husband.

Narrowing the Egg Donor Search

Many fertility clinics will assist couples in finding a donor egg or provide referrals to agencies that deal with the testing, evaluation and screening of donors. Clinics and agencies have strict guidelines and acceptance criteria when determining their donor registry. While the standards may vary, with proper research you can find an agency that will locate a donor who will meet or even exceed your expectations. In addition to your fertility clinic, the ASRM is a key resource that you can use to understand and gather information regarding egg donors and other third-party reproductive options.

The genetic and medical screening an egg donor goes through is a complicated process and comprised of many layers. The donor's family medical history is screened for birth defects, genetic disorders and mental illnesses. In addition, the donor herself undergoes a complete physical examination as well as a formal psychological evaluation. Finally, she must undergo testing for any sexually transmitted diseases.

Donors are also classified by age and ethnic background. The ASRM recommends that, in general, donors should be younger than thirty-five years, with no history of infertility, and all tests should reflect a normal ovarian reserve. Some agencies cap their donor egg age at twenty-nine, and most require a minimum age of twenty-one; however, there are some agencies that will work with donors as young as nineteen. Are you wondering where these young, spry candidates come from? Many agencies target universities and college campuses to find prospective donors.

Some agencies offer you a two-tier donation program. The more conventional group offers donors who meet baseline criteria, weighing heavily in favor of physical resemblance and high scores on standardized tests and those who pass all medical screening. The second-tier (read: more selective) offers the same criteria as well as intellectual aptitude. The second-tier donors are required to have both an undergraduate and a graduate degree, high SAT scores or a grade point average of 3.50. If some of you are reeling right now realizing that your *own* eggs wouldn't be in the extraordinary tier, don't feel bad; we're convinced ours would be in the previously viewed, semi-used, half-price bin.

Using a fertility clinic or an agency to secure your donor egg may not be right for you. You may seek your options privately. Many couples prefer to find their own source and solicit donors via the World Wide Web. One of our TTCs made the decision to seek an egg donor and began a private search. She and her husband began receiving cards and letters filled with pictures of women and their personal profiles. While our TTC was in search of a donor who was smart and looked like her, her husband seemed more interested in finding a donor who looked great in a bikini. If going the egg donor route, save yourself time and arguments by establishing the donor criteria with your husband before you begin the search.

Your Nest Egg

You've done it; you've found the perfect match. Your donor passed all the required prescreening tests, and you feel confident she's the one. You're anxious to move on to the actual egg donation process. In the back of your mind, you've made a mental note to tuck away approximately $5,000 to $7,000 in the "expense department" for the egg donor fee. But before making a commitment, it's time to examine the procedures and costs more closely. The $5,000 to $7,000 can be deceiving, as it only covers the actual donor compensation portion of the transfer. A typical fee schedule can vary but will most likely include donor screening charges, donor cycle fees, recipient cycle fees, donor transfer fees, donor insurance, anesthesia, donor medications and your IVF cycle—all totaling a whopping $40,000.

Using a donor egg can be a tough decision for couples to make and certainly one that needs thorough consideration. Because there are no guarantees and the associated costs are so high, it's often a hard decision to make. The pregnancy success rates depend on many factors, but in the latest statistic available (1993 SART report), the overall live birth rate for donor egg programs was 30 percent per transfer; however, rates do vary considerably from program to program.

I'd Like to Make a Withdrawal: Donor Sperm

Rarely discussed in this book (or on the golf course) is the topic of male infertility. Couples who experience male infertility, without any female fertility issues, may decide donor sperm is an option.

Before moving to donor insemination (DI), however, couples experiencing male infertility may want to consider a relatively new treatment procedure called intracytoplasmic sperm injection

(ICSI). Through the advancement of technology, doctors are now able to inject a single sperm into an egg, causing fertilization. This process is used to help couples when the male has a very low sperm count or poor motility. By hand-selecting the best sperm, a couple's chance of success greatly increases.

For more severe male infertility factors, ICSI may not be an option; however, couples can still maintain half the biological tie through the use of donor sperm. Male infertility issues are just as distressing as female issues, and men will also need to mourn the loss of a biological connection to their children should they choose to use donor sperm. Although most men don't wear their hearts on their sleeves, be sensitive to the fact that your husband may be silently suffering because he is unable to get you pregnant.

The donor sperm procedure is much less complicated than using donor eggs. Basically, the woman undergoes an IUI at the time of ovulation, using the donor's sperm instead of her husband's. According to RESOLVE, 60 to 80 percent of couples who use donor sperm achieve pregnancy; however, it may take many cycles.

Finding donor sperm isn't quite as complicated as finding donor eggs, primarily because frozen semen is more readily available, and there are sperm banks that offer anonymous donors. Couples have a choice as to which sperm bank and which donor they will use, but much like finding a donor egg, it is important that the bank screen the donors medically as well as provide pertinent information such as physical characteristics, race, ethnic background and educational/career history. General health profiles must include HIV test results as well as any other sexually transmitted diseases.

It's not uncommon for sperm banks to provide photographs of donors, so here's your chance to have a little fun. You can select a donor with the looks of a J. Crew model and the intellect of a Harvard Business School grad.

If you're considering using donor sperm, an excellent resource for gathering details about sperm banks is the American Foundation for Urologic Disease (*www.afud.org*). Another resource featuring sperm bank information is the American Association of Tissue Banks (*www.aatb.org*).

The Big Chill: Donor Embryos

Couples who suffer from both male and female fertility issues may pursue the option of a donor embryo. While this may seem like an extreme option, donor embryos allow the experience of childbirth for women who are capable of carrying a baby to term, but who cannot get pregnant with her own eggs and her husband's sperm. Essentially, if implantation and uterine problems are not the cause of female infertility, then embryo donation may be a good solution.

According to a 2003 report by SART and the nonprofit research institution RAND Corporation, approximately 400,000 embryos are cryopreserved (frozen) in the United States. Many of the embryos in storage are the unused embryos that remain from couples who have completed their families through IVF. These couples may choose to donate their remaining embryos to another couple rather than having them destroyed or donated to scientific research.

You can find an embryo donor a variety of ways. The first, and perhaps most common, is an anonymous donation through an IVF clinic. Upon consultation, the clinic will try to match a couple with an embryo using physical characteristics and ethnicity. The medical evaluation for donor embryos is much the same as any other third-party reproductive criteria, requiring all of the medical and psychological screening as well as testing for any sexually transmitted diseases.

In an open donation, the couple donating the embryo will take an active role in the selection of the couple intended to receive the embryo, much like in an open adoption. The process actually allows a donor to consider the recipient's ethnic background, income and education. Another scenario has the donor playing a less active role in the selection process, but the donor is still informed if a birth results. The donor may want to establish a relationship with the recipient couple after the birth of the baby. If this is the case, all factors should be considered both from a legal and an emotional standpoint. Clearly, these are exceptional circumstances, and the decision will need to be made while taking into consideration how much contact the donor couple will have with the recipient and baby.

It's important to remember that while some of these options are a fundamental departure from what you imagined for your family, they can still fulfill your dream of having a child. One of our TTCs almost fell off her chair while, over a latte, one of her best friends, who had been successful with IVF, offered our TTC one of her own frozen embryos. Not surprisingly, our TTC misheard her friend and struggled to make sense of the proposition, wondering, "Did she just offer me an AM radio? Why would I need an AM radio?" After quickly realizing what her friend had said, our TTC thought it the kindest gesture she had ever experienced. And although she declined, she was moved and amazed at her friend's humbling generosity.

According to the CDC, the birth rate for frozen donor embryo transfer is less than 24 percent. Not surprising, given so many factors play a role. As opposed to egg donors, who are screened for age, medical history and intellectual aptitude, embryo donors could have reduced egg quality and fertility issues of their own.

The costs for frozen embryo donation can include preparation of cryopreserved embryos for transfer, ultrasounds, assisted hatching and IVF—for the daunting total of nearly $30,000.

There are no easy answers when dealing with third-party reproduction. Each couple must consider their individual feelings when faced with making decisions about building their family with the help of a genetic donor. Conflicting feelings are to be expected, and couples may have very different opinions about what the "right" thing to do is. By allowing time to work through the alternatives before committing to a solution, the joys of motherhood may still be an option by embracing the available opportunities.

Womb for Rent: Surrogate Mothers

Infertility comes in all shapes and sizes, but it has one thing in common—there's a wake of heartbreak and emotional exhaustion behind every diagnosis. Some couples are lulled into a state of relief when they are easily able to get pregnant, only to have their happiness shattered over and over again when they are unable to carry the pregnancy to term. There are many medical reasons why a woman may not be able to successfully carry a baby full term. For those couples who hold on to the dream of a biological child, there is still hope with the help of a surrogate mother.

Although certainly not mainstream, the use of surrogate mothers has been somewhat demystified, thanks in part to Kelsey Grammer and his wife, Camille, and Joan Lunden and her husband, Jeff Konigsberg. Celebrities are not the only ones turning to surrogates to help realize their dreams of a family. According to the Organization of Parents Through Surrogacy (OPTS), a nonprofit organization dedicated to providing support and information on surrogacy, there have been more than 10,000 babies born to surrogate mothers in the United States since the 1970s.

Before deciding if a surrogate is right for you, take some time to consider your individual situation, and have a serious discussion with your husband to gauge each other's comfort levels with surrogacy versus other family-building options.

Once you and your husband agree surrogacy is the right choice, it's critical to do some investigating and learn everything you can about the available resources. OPTS is a good first stop (*www.opts.com*). The organization offers networking services to put you in touch with the professional resources you need as well as introduces you to other couples who have already been through the process. Creating a network of support with those who have lived through a surrogate arrangement will be a lifeline for advice and information.

Because surrogacy is an unregulated industry, you will find drastic discrepancies in the quality of resources available. A quick cruise down the information superhighway will reveal everything from agencies in luxury high-rises promising you the uber-surrogate to snapshots of a woman in her living room offering her services for a quick three-hundred bucks. If a deal sounds too good to be true, it probably is.

What Exactly Is a Surrogate?

There are two basic types of surrogacy. The traditional surrogate mother is inseminated with the intended father's sperm via an IUI. The father's sperm unites with the surrogate's egg to create the embryo, making the surrogate both the biological as well as the birth mother.

The second option is *gestational surrogacy*. In this case, the intended parents go through IVF, and their embryo is then implanted in the surrogate. The surrogate, also referred to as the gestational carrier or host uterus, acts as the birth mother but has no genetic tie to the child. The baby is 100 percent the genetic offspring of the couple. If there are male fertility issues, the couple may opt to use the intended mother's eggs and donor sperm, or if there are female issues, the couple may use the intended father's sperm along with donor eggs.

Parental rights via surrogacy vary by state and therefore must be addressed prior to entering into an agreement. The last thing you want is a drawn-out legal process to establish custody after the baby is born, so be sure to review both your state laws, as well as your surrogate's state laws, in detail with your attorney.

Is There a Surrogate in the House?

When faced with the challenge of finding a surrogate, many couples turn to family or friends. These couples take comfort knowing their precious cargo will be in good hands for the next nine months, and in the case of a sister, there's the added benefit the baby will be nurtured by the closest genetic equivalent of his or her biological mother.

One night, a group of our friends got together for dinner at a local Mexican restaurant. As a festive mariachi band filled the room with music, a late-arriving friend flew through the door and cha cha cha'd over to the table, clearly sporting a pregnant belly. She already had two small children, but we had no idea she was considering a third. When the chorus of congratulations started, she quickly cut everyone off and said, "Oh, it's not mine." The impossible happened. Six women fell speechless as their minds raced to process the information. Before we had a chance to bombard her with questions, she quickly announced she was acting as a surrogate, carrying her sister's child. When she told us her husband was not only supportive but that it was originally his idea, we unanimously pronounced them the two most caring people in the universe and toasted them with frozen margaritas (virgin for her). Truly, what greater gift can one human give to another?

If your sister's uterus is not available or you'd rather not involve your close friends and family, there are plenty of caring women out there who are ready, willing and able to help you with your dreams of motherhood. You may wonder what the motivation is behind becoming a surrogate mother. In some cases, it may be financially driven, but in other cases, it is truly a calling.

One of our TTCs told us that her surrogate mother was told at an early age she would never be able to have children. Understanding the pain of infertility firsthand, she decided to become a surrogate after she proved "them" wrong by successfully building her own family.

How does one find a surrogate mother? There are basically two ways: you can either seek the help of a surrogate agency, or you can choose to go it on your own. If you choose to work independently, there are a host of Web sites available to put you in touch with potential surrogate mothers. Again, be sure to get recommendations for high-quality sites with good reputations.

To avoid scams and to ease the burden of the process, many couples opt to go with a professional surrogate agency. The agency is typically responsible for screening potential candidates, finding a suitable match, managing the contracts, handling the financial aspects and acting as an intermediary should problems arise. Of course, nothing in life is free, and according to OPTS, agencies charge anywhere from $8,000 to $15,000 for their services.

Shopping for a Surrogate

So just what should you consider when searching for the woman who is going to carry your baby? Of course, the most obvious and important thing you want is someone who is in good health, both mentally and physically. Aside from the medical considerations, many of the other qualities you will look for in a surrogate will be personal preference. For some couples, it's extremely important for the surrogate to have prior experience, while others are comfortable with a first-timer. Other considerations, which may be important to you, include whether the surrogate smokes, drinks alcohol, eats healthy foods, exercises, likes pets, lives in the same state and so on. As you move through the search, you may find you are willing to bend on some issues, while others are a deal breaker.

How Much for the Blonde?

Just how much does a surrogate go for these days? Women consider price comparison an Olympic sport. Whether it's a designer pair of sling-backs discovered at rock-bottom prices at the Designer Shoe Warehouse or the inflated cost of avocados after a spell of bad weather, women want to know that they're getting a good deal. As you've traveled along the road of fertility treatment, you may have been lucky enough to have a friend in the same boat who could serve as your blue book for medical costs. Saturday-morning calls skipped the pleasantries and got right to the issue: "Can you believe my doctor charges $150 for an office visit?" "That's nothing," your friend replied. "My doctor charges $200, and he barely says ten words. That's twenty bucks a word." Once again, you felt better as you looked at the stack of medical bills piled on your desk, not because you thought they were reasonable, but because you realized you weren't the only one being ripped off by a guy in a white coat.

Odds are, however, you're probably going to be on your own when exploring the cost of a surrogate mother. The sheer cost of surrogacy can be a bit overwhelming, and the degree to which the estimates vary make it all the more confusing. This is where your new circle of surrogate friends comes in. The support organizations, as well as couples who have already been through the experience, can tell you if something sounds unreasonably high or too good to be true.

When we called agents looking for surrogacy estimates, they said, "Whatever you think it's going to cost, add another twenty percent." The cost of using a surrogate can vary widely, depending on the individual situation, but on average, the total cost is in the range of $45,000 to $60,000. However, it can go as high as $100,000. A couple may be quoted a surrogate fee of $15,000 to $35,000, but they must remember that they are responsible for all of the medical expenses for both themselves and the surrogate throughout the process. A typical contract allows for three attempted pregnancies, which means the extra cost of three IVFs if using a gestational carrier. Whatever the final cost may be, remember, this woman is taking nine months of her life to change yours forever.

The Adoption Option

Some children are born from their mother's belly; others are born from their mother's heart. Whether you've decided not to venture down the path of fertility treatment or been battered along the way, you may at some point find yourself contemplating adoption to help you build your family. Many couples look at adoption as their final chance at parenthood, only after exhausting all potential medical avenues. Others actively discuss adoption early on in their efforts to conceive because they know assisted reproduction is not a viable option for them. And then there are couples who, while they may be able to get pregnant on their own, have always dreamed of adopting a child.

For couples who have repeatedly been unsuccessful at conceiving—with or without fertility treatment—adoption may not be an immediate consideration for them. Yet one day, they open their hearts and minds to adoption. Perhaps it was a failed final IVF attempt, a heartbreaking miscarriage or the ultimate acceptance that they will never give birth to a child of their own. Regardless of what serves as the inspiration, adopting a child can be one of the most rewarding experiences of your life. With adoption, both the parents and the children win. Couples who desperately want to be loving parents are connected with children who need a family.

Where Do You Begin?

The fact is, it doesn't matter how or when you come to your decision to adopt a child. Once you get there, you will feel an unbelievable surge of energy and excitement to begin the process of finding your baby and building your family. Only after you and your husband are completely comfortable with your decision to adopt does the real work begin. Be prepared for a complicated, over-whelming and sometimes frustrating process. Like every major endeavor you've faced together, adoption will require you to do your homework.

You know there are many decisions you will have to make when considering what kind of adoption you want to pursue. However, you may not even know what questions to begin asking to get things in motion. To help set your course, visit the National Adoption Information Clearinghouse Web site (*http://naic.acf.hhs.gov*). Sponsored by the U.S. Department of Health and Human Services, the NAIC is a comprehensive resource on all aspects of adoption. Their Web site provides a wealth of information and valuable links that will help answer the multitude of questions you are sure to have, including baseline adoption statistics; the variety of adoption options from which to choose (domestic or international, agency or independent); information to help locate local agencies and sup-port groups; the average costs of adoption; federal and state adop-tion laws, including waiting periods and consent; as well as information for accessing adoption records, recommended books for children and adoption-related conferences.

Don't fret. Once you've sorted through the basics, you will more clearly understand the long and winding road you'll need to navigate in the adoption process.

Born in the USA: Domestic Adoption

One of the first questions you are likely to ask yourself is whether you are interested in a domestic or international adoption. If you determine you are interested in adopting a child born stateside, there is then the choice to make between adopting through an independent adoption (typically arranged through an attorney or facilitator) or an agency adoption (public or private).

Independent Adoption: Attorney or Facilitator

In an independent adoption, the adopting parents typically locate the birth parents on their own with the help of their attorney or facilitator. The NAIC estimates that families who pursue independent adoptions can expect to spend anywhere from $8,000 to $30,000. Costs may include, but are not limited to, attorney fees for you and possibly the birth mother, advertising associated with finding a birth mother, pregnancy-related medical expenses, living expenses, home study and other costs, such as counseling for you and/or the birth mother.

An attorney's role in an idependent adoption can vary widely from simply navigating the complex legal system to acting more like an agency and handling most aspects of the adoption, including locating a birth mother. Before you commit to working with a specific attorney, make sure you do some investigating to be certain he or she specializes in adoption and doesn't just practice it on the side when not chasing ambulances or defending shoplifters. Adoption laws vary widely, and you want an attorney who is experienced and knows how to best work within the laws of your state. Attorney's fees vary, based on their level of involvement in the adoption, but you can expect the fees to be anywhere from $8,000 to $15,000.

Another alternative in an independent adoption is to use an adoption facilitator. A facilitator is someone who works with a couple to find a birth mother and charges a fee for their services, which can range from $4,000 to $8,000. While the facilitator will handle all aspects of locating a birth mother, you will still need to contract an attorney to handle the legal aspects, and you'll need to work with a licensed agency to conduct a home study.

According to NAIC, facilitators are now allowed in most states; however, they are not usually state licensed or regulated by any government agency. So if you choose to work with a facilitator, make sure he or she has plenty of experience—and the references to prove it.

If you are interested in adopting an infant, an independent adoption may be the right choice for you. Many attorneys and facilitators specialize in newborn adoptions. Of course, there are always exceptions, but the time it typically takes to find an infant through an independent adoption can be much less than if you were working with an agency.

Agency Adoption: Public or Private

If you determine agency adoption is preferred over an attorney or facilitator adoption, you will then have to choose between a state/public agency or a private adoption agency.

Children available for adoption at public agencies have been taken into state custody due to parental mistreatment or neglect, because they have been orphaned or because their parents can no longer take care of them. These children are often referred to as wards of the state. Often, the children also have siblings in custody, and the state will try its best to keep the family together through temporary foster family care. Many children remain in foster care for years with the hope that the agency will one day be able to return the children to their parents. However, if at any point the state terminates the parental rights of the birth parents, the children will become eligible for adoption.

Public agency adoption is typically much less expensive than private agency adoption, and some states offer subsidies to adoptive families to help defray the costs associated with raising the children. According to the NAIC, public adoption expenses range from zero to $2,500, including travel and attorney's fees. If you are interested in pursuing public adoption, a good place to begin your research is to call or visit the Web site for your local Division of Youth and Family Services (DYFS) or whatever the comparable agency may be referred to in your state.

If you wish to adopt an infant, you will most likely choose to work with a private agency, because state agencies tend to have older children or those with special needs. Private agencies are licensed by the state in which they perform their business, and they must abide by the adoption laws of that state. Unlike an independent adoption, a private agency handles all aspects of the adoption, so you won't need to outsource any additional services.

Be aware that many private agencies have specific criteria for infant adoption, and it is important to understand what these criteria are up front. Ask if the agency has age, marital history or employment requirements for the adopting parents. Some agencies may only consider couples between the ages of twenty-five and forty, who have been married for at least three years and who can show a stable income. Find out whether the agency limits its adoptions to couples who cannot bear children on their own or to couples who currently have no other children. If you are a dual-income household, ask if the agency allows both parents to work outside of the home immediately following the adoption.

According to the NAIC, a domestic private agency adoption can range from $4,000 to $30,000. Some agencies have sliding fee scales based on family income. But remember, before you make a commitment to work with any agency, make sure their license is current; if it's not, there's probably a reason why, and you'll want to know what it is.

Passport and Boarding Pass Required: International Adoption

International adoptions are on the rise in the United States. Every year, more and more couples are looking oversees to find a child to call their own. There are many reasons why couples decide on international adoption over domestic. Cost is typically *not* one of them. According to the NAIC, fees for intercountry adoption can range from $7,000 to $25,000, including agency fees, dossier and immigration processing fees and court costs. Additional costs you may incur include the home study fee (done by a different agency if the international agency is based in another state), travel and in-country stays to process the adoption abroad (length of stay or number of visits may vary), escorting fees (charged when you do not travel but instead hire escorts to accompany the child on the flight to your country) and, in some countries, the child's medical care and treatment.

When considering international adoption, many couples think the process to adopt an infant will be easier than if they were to adopt domestically. However, after seeing the abundance of paperwork required and the bureaucratic red tape they will endure, they might quickly change their opinions. Since the process can take longer than a domestic adoption, babies are somewhat older (six to twelve months) by the time you are able to take them home.

Some couples are inspired to adopt internationally because they see it as an act of compassion to help children who they believe have been mistreated by their government or culture. In the 1970s, Americans adopted thousands of South Korean and Vietnamese children. Adoptions of Chinese girls have skyrocketed in the past decade as reports surfaced that Chinese orphanages were overflowing with baby girls because of the country's cultural preference for boys. Many children have also been adopted from orphanages in war-torn countries in the former Soviet Union and Romania.

No matter your personal reason for choosing international adoption, once you are ready to move ahead, you will take many of the same steps you would in a domestic adoption as well as a few extras added along the way. Be prepared—it is a much more complicated process because you are dealing with two different countries, each with its own adoption laws. Due to the complexities involved in international adoption, the most important step you will take is to find a reputable international agency that can help you navigate the labyrinth that lies ahead.

There are several Web sites that can be helpful in beginning your international adoption search. Check out International Adoption (*www.internationaladoption.org*), the U.S. Citizenship and Immigration Services (*www.uscis.gov*) and the Web site run by the U.S. Department of State (*www.travel.state.gov/family*). These sites offer an abundance of information about the various countries that offer international adoption programs. The USCIS page can provide you with the official forms that you will need to complete as part of your adoption dossier.

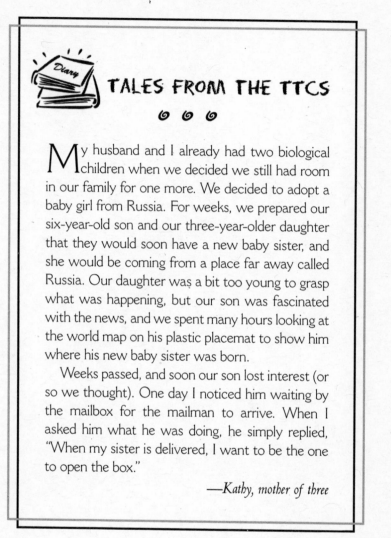

TALES FROM THE TTCS

🌀 🌀 🌀

My husband and I already had two biological children when we decided we still had room in our family for one more. We decided to adopt a baby girl from Russia. For weeks, we prepared our six-year-old son and our three-year-older daughter that they would soon have a new baby sister, and she would be coming from a place far away called Russia. Our daughter was a bit too young to grasp what was happening, but our son was fascinated with the news, and we spent many hours looking at the world map on his plastic placemat to show him where his new baby sister was born.

Weeks passed, and soon our son lost interest (or so we thought). One day I noticed him waiting by the mailbox for the mailman to arrive. When I asked him what he was doing, he simply replied, "When my sister is delivered, I want to be the one to open the box."

—*Kathy, mother of three*

chapter fourteen

Mama, Madre, Mommy, Mum

Thursday	Notes

- *Buy pregnancy tests*

Friday	Notes	Saturday	Notes

mother (mŭth'ər)

n. *A woman who conceives, gives birth to, or raises and nurtures a child.*

Just When You Least Expect It

You can't take it one more minute. Today's the day you find out if you're pregnant. As you let your mind wander in the land of plush pink and blue baby blankets, you decide you just can't wait for the late-afternoon call from the doctor's office with the results of your pregnancy test. You have to know now. You jump in the car and head to the drugstore to purchase a pregnancy kit—not the entire store shelf, just a single box with two sticks.

Not wanting to watch the window of the test deny you motherhood once again, you leave the room. Upon returning *exactly* two minutes later (some things never change), you see them—the double pink lines! You quickly unwrap and take the second test. The results are the same—YOU ARE PREGNANT!

You've waited months (possibly years) for this day to come, and now you stand in your bathroom both laughing and crying at the same time. You are thrilled, relieved and overwhelmed with emotion. You grab the test and run to the backyard to find your husband, who's mowing the lawn. You wave your arms wildly trying to get his attention while firmly grasping the stick, not wanting to let it go. When he finally sees you, he stops and, despite the bright afternoon sun, looks at you with wide-open eyes. He knows something is either terribly wrong or wonderfully right. As he walks closer, it takes every ounce of energy to contain the excitement you feel. You want to scream out, "I'm pregnant!" but instead, you wait until he is standing in front of you, looking both scared and hopeful. You gently kiss him on the cheek, place the test in his hands and tell him he is going to be a father. Through tears and laughter, you embrace and revel in the moment—you are going to have a baby.

To: Courtney <Courtney@conceptionchronicles.com>;
          Shelly <Shelly@conceptionchronicles.com>
From: Patty <Patty@conceptionchronicles.com>
Subject: **I can't believe it . . .**

I'm PREGNANT!!!! I'm in complete shock. After all this time, I wasn't sure it would ever happen. Scott and I are out of our minds.

To: Patty <Patty@conceptionchronicles.com>
From: Courtney <Courtney@conceptionchronicles.com>
Cc: Shelly <Shelly@conceptionchronicles.com>
Subject: **OH MY GOD!**

CONGRATULATIONS!!!! This is incredible. I just got your message on my Blackberry. I'm in a cab with a client, and I started to cry. Thank God it's a woman! I'm so thrilled for you guys. I'll call you tonight.

To: Patty <Patty@conceptionchronicles.com>
From: Shelly <Shelly@conceptionchronicles.com>
Cc: Courtney <Courtney@conceptionchronicles.com>
Subject: **RE: OH MY GOD!**

CONGRATULATIONS!!!! I'm screaming so loud you can probably hear me all the way in Connecticut!! I wish I was there to give you a gigantic hug. Maybe you will get the summer off after all. I'll call you later—I'm dying to talk to you.

Pinch Me, Please

You may feel a little numb when you finally see the double pink lines or receive the call from the doctor's office that starts with "Congratulations" instead of the dreaded "I'm sorry" you've grown accustomed to hearing. You expected to feel pure joy, and while you are out of your mind with excitement, there may also be a twinge of anxiety hanging in the air. You've waited for this moment for so long—you just hope everything is going to be okay.

Welcome to motherhood. From this day forward, you will worry about your baby and question your ability to be a good mother. While this is perfectly normal, don't let your fears spoil the excitement of your pregnancy. As for your fears of motherhood, every woman has them. You have a lifetime to perfect that which you have joyously struggled to achieve—being a mother.

Where There's a Will There's a Way

In taking an alternative path to motherhood, you didn't diminish the remarkable journey—you created a new road to your ultimate destination. The amazing news may have been delivered in the pink lines from a pregnancy test stick or a meeting with a surrogate mother. The fact is, there is more than one road to motherhood.

Whether your baby passes through your birth canal or international customs, when he or she is placed into your arms for the first time, the joy that overwhelms you will dissolve any pain it took to get you there.

The Ties That Bind

Your fertility journey has taught you commitment—to yourself, to your spouse and to your future son or daughter. When you initially embarked on your quest to have a child, you and your husband were linked with the promise of creating a family. While your path took unexpected twists and turns, and some corners were filled with doubt, in the end, your love for each other and your dedication fulfilled your dream.

There were times you felt alone and that not a soul could understand what you were going through. Then it would happen: a hug from your husband after your evening shot or his secretly returning your wedding band to your finger while you were still in a haze recovering from surgery; a funny e-mail from your girlfriend to lift you up after each failed attempt or a call from your mother offering her unwaivering support and a hand delivery of your favorite homemade cookies. These are the gestures, the shared experiences that bind you for life.

You have no idea what lies ahead with pregnancy, never mind motherhood (and your husband is probably more in the dark than you). But you are certain you are ready to face the challenges along the way—especially with the frontline support from your girlfriends who have ventured into motherhood before you.

Congratulations, Mom.

Epilogue

Three Months Later . . .

To:	Courtney <Courtney@conceptionchronicles.com>;
	Shelly <Shelly@conceptionchronicles.com>
From:	Patty <Patty@conceptionchronicles.com>
Subject:	**You've got to be kidding me.**

You're going to die when you see the new full-figured me. I finally have cleavage, but now suddenly my skin has turned to Saran Wrap. You can practically see the blood running through my veins.

It's the ultimate irony. I finally have something to show off, but nobody would want to see it.

To:	Patty <Patty@conceptionchronicles.com>
From:	Courtney <Courtney@conceptionchronicles.com>
Cc:	Shelly <Shelly@conceptionchronicles.com>
Subject:	**RE: You've got to be kidding me.**

I remember when I had to upgrade to a maternity bra. My boobs were HUGE, but they were killing me. Dan said it was like getting a new car and not being allowed to drive it.

To:	Patty <Patty@conceptionchronicles.com>;
	Courtney <Courtney@conceptionchronicles.com>
From:	Shelly <Shelly@conceptionchronicles.com>
Subject:	**More to come . . .**

Just wait. Pregnancy brings all sorts of surprises . . . some more pleasant than others.

To:	Patty <Patty@conceptionchronicles.com>;
	Shelly <Shelly@conceptionchronicles.com>
From:	Courtney <Courtney@conceptionchronicles.com>
Subject:	**The best surprise of all . . .**

Like the first time you feel the baby kick. I'll remember that feeling for the rest of my life!

To:	Shelly <Shelly@conceptionchronicles.com>;
	Courtney <Courtney@conceptionchronicles.com>
From:	Patty <Patty@conceptionchronicles.com>
Subject:	**I can't wait . . .**

Until I really look pregnant, and I can feel the baby move, I still won't believe it—it just doesn't seem real.

To:	Patty <Patty@conceptionchronicles.com>;
	Courtney <Courtney@conceptionchronicles.com>
From:	Shelly <Shelly@conceptionchronicles.com>
Subject:	**Pace yourself**

Just let it all soak in. You're given nine months for a reason.

To:	Patty <Patty@conceptionchronicles.com>;
	Shelly <Shelly@conceptionchronicles.com>
From:	Courtney <Courtney@conceptionchronicles.com>
Subject:	**RE: Pace yourself**

Shelly's right—your pregnancy will be a blur, and once the baby's born you'll barely remember your life before.

To: Patty <Patty@conceptionchronicles.com>;
           Courtney <Courtney@conceptionchronicles.com>
From: Shelly <Shelly@conceptionchronicles.com>
Subject: **What life before??**

And you can't even imagine the love you're going to feel. I remember people telling me that when I was pregnant, but I never really understood until I held Maré in my arms.

To: Shelly <Shelly@conceptionchronicles.com>;
           Courtney <Courtney@conceptionchronicles.com>
From: Patty <Patty@conceptionchronicles.com>
Subject: **RE: What life before??**

I couldn't have made it this far without you girls. It's so good to know you'll be here for the next six months.

To: Patty <Patty@conceptionchronicles.com>;
           Shelly <Shelly@conceptionchronicles.com>
From: Courtney <Courtney@conceptionchronicles.com>
Subject: **Of course we're here for the next six months . . .**

And the next 18 years!!

For a list of fertility resources, updates from the authors (did Patty have a boy or a girl?) and more, please visit:

www.conceptionchronicles.com

To post an online fertility journal (your own "Conception Chronicle!") and discuss the "ovulation olympics", "fertile friends and foes", "sex on demand", and other topics inspired by this book, please visit the iVillage conception chronicles community forum at:

www.ivillage.com/conceptionchronicles

Resources

Fertility-Related Organizations

The American College of Obstetricians and Gynecologists: 409 12th Street, S.W., PO Box 96920, Washington, D.C. 20090-6920. Telephone: (202) 638-5577. *www.acog.org*

American Society of Reproductive Medicine: 1209 Montgomery Highway, Birmingham, Alabama 35216-2809. Telephone: (205) 978-5000. Fax: (205) 978-5005. *www.asrm.org*

Centers for Disease Control and Prevention: 1600 Clifton Road, Atlanta, Georgia 30333. Telephone: (404) 639-3311/ Public Inquiries: (404) 639-3534/(800) 311-3435. *www.CDC.gov*

The International Council on Infertility Information Dissemination (INCIID): PO Box 6836, Arlington, Virginia 22206. Telephone: (703) 379-9178. Fax: (703) 379-1593. *www.inciid.org*

LifebankUSA: Provides umbilical cord blood banking services for families, 45 Horsehill Road, Cedar Knolls, New Jersey 07927. Telephone: (877) 543-3226 or *LifebankUSA.com.*

RAND Corporation: 1776 Main Street, PO Box 2138, Santa Monica, California 90407-2138. Telephone: (310) 393-0411. Fax: (310) 393-4818. *www.rand.org*

RESOLVE: The National Infertility Association: 7910 Woodmont Avenue, Suite 1350, Bethesda, Maryland 20814. Telephone: (301) 652-8585. Fax: (301) 652-9375. *www.resolve.org*

The American Fertility Association (AFA): 666 Fifth Avenue, Suite 278, New York, New York 10103. Telephone: (888) 917-3777. Fax: (718) 601-7722. *www.theafa.org*

Society for Assisted Reproductive Technology: Contact Joyce Zeitz, Executive Administrator, 1209 Montgomery Highway, Birmingham, Alabama 35216. Telephone: (205) 978-5000, ext. 109. Fax: (205) 978-5015. *www.sart.org*

Fertility-Related Web Sites

www.babycenter.com This is the go-to site for everything baby. Plus there are great chat rooms and bulletin board postings for everyone in every situation.

www.fertilityfriend.com Offers tools for tracking ovulation, pinpointing fertile days and basal body temperature chart analysis.

www.fertilitylifelines.com Created by Serono, Inc., the site provides information on infertility and treatment options.

www.fertilityneighborhood.com A service of Freedom Drug. A resource for treatment options, insurance coverage issues and information about fertility drugs.

www.FocusOnFertility.org A newsletter provided by the American Fertility Association and Organon USA, Inc. Covers all topics related to male and female infertility.

www.gettingpregnant.co.uk Offers information on all the basics of getting pregnant along with a side of British wit.

www.ivfconnections.com This site is obviously for those who are seeking fertility treatment, but even those not going through IVF will find interesting information. Features IVF bulletin boards.

www.iVillage.com A resource for women, containing many articles on pregnancy and fertility.

www.labtestsonline.org Lab Tests Online is a public resource, which provides information regarding fertility blood tests.

Male Fertility—Related Web Sites

www.afud.org American Foundation for Urologic Disease. Information on all topics related to men's health.

www.aatb.org The American Association of Tissue Banks. Provides information and resources for finding donor sperm.

www.maleinfertility.com Sponsored by Cornell University—Weill Medical College—Cornell Institute for Reproductive Medicine. Provides useful resources for all issues related to male infertility.

Books on Fertility

Fertility for Dummies by Jackie Meyers-Thompson and Sharon Perkins, R.N. Explores the path of infertility from trying to conceive to high-tech treatments.

Taking Charge of Your Fertility: The Definitive Guide to Natural Birth Control, Pregnancy Achievement, and Reproductive Health by Toni Weschler. This book is the encyclopedia of all that is female and answers the most basic questions about your menstrual cycle to the more daunting concerns around assisted reproduction.

The Infertility Cure: The Ancient Chinese Wellness Program for Getting Pregnant and Having Healthy Babies by Randine Lewis, Ph.D. A resource for women seeking to boost their chances of pregnancy through Chinese medicine.

Third-Party Reproduction

www.conceptualoptions.com Conceptual Options—Partnering for Parenthood Through Surrogacy and Egg Donation. A good first stop when considering third-party reproduction.

www.opts.com The Organization of Parents Through Surrogacy. A nationally recognized nonprofit surrogacy support organization providing services to the surrogacy community.

Adoption

Adoption for Dummies by Tracy Barr and Katrina Carlisle. The complete resource for domestic and international adoption.

www.internationaladoption.org Provides everything from basic questions about selecting a particular country, age restrictions, dossiers, and referrals to welcoming your child.

http://naic.acf.hhs.gov National Adoption Information Clearinghouse (NAIC): Offers national adoption directory search, state-by-state licensed adoption agencies, support groups and more.

www.travel.state.gov/family Sponsored by the U.S. Department of State. The Overseas Citizens Services (OCS) works with a wide range of domestic and international organizations to assist American citizen families in the United States and abroad.

www.uscis.gov The U.S. Citizenship and Immigration Services offers information concerning international adoption.

About the Authors

After battling infertility for three years, Patty Doyle Debano is pregnant with her first child. She lives in Connecticut with her husband, Scott, and their slightly overweight golden retriever. Courtney Edgerton Menzel is the mother of a daughter, five, and a son, three. She lives in Chicago with her husband, Dan, and manages to balance the demands of motherhood and a full-time career thanks to a variety of take-out menus. Shelly Dicken Sutphen is the mother of a "spirited" three-year-old daughter. She lives in San Diego with her husband, Bruce, and, surprisingly, has the energy to try for number two.

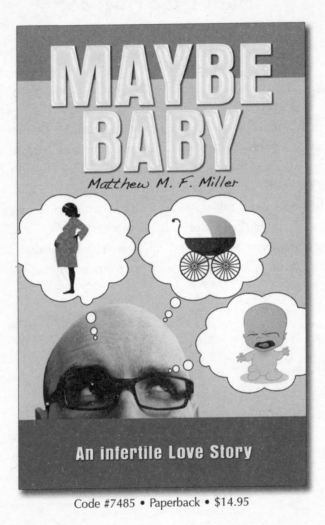